Traditional Acupuncture: The Law of the Five Elements

Also by Dianne M. Connelly

All Sickness is Home Sickness

and
two new books tentatively titled *Lovers*
and *Alive and Awake* will be published soon.

Traditional Acupuncture: The Law of the Five Elements

Dianne M. Connelly, Ph.D., M.Ac.

Cover Design by John C. Wilson
Cover Photograph by Kathleen Thormod Carr, © 1991
Author Photograph by Walter Larrimore
Art by John Levering

Library of Congress Cataloging

Connelly, Dianne M., 1945–
    Traditional acupuncture: the law of the five elements/Dianne M. Connelly.—2nd ed.
        p. cm
    Includes bibliographical references and index.
    ISBN 0-912381-03-5: $16.00
    1. Acupuncture.   2. Medicine, Chinese.   I. Title.
RM184.C66   1994
615.8'92—dc20   94-39074
                                                                CIP

Grateful acknowledgment is made for permission to reprint excerpts from the following works:

The lines from "if everything happens that can't be done" are reprinted from COMPLETE POEMS, 1904–1962, by E.E. Cummings, Edited by George J. Firmage, by permission of Liveright Publishing Corporation. Copyright © 1944, 1972, 1991 by the Trustees for the E.E. Cummings Trust.

Octavio Paz: Configurations. Copyright © 1971 by New Directions Publishing Corporation. Reprinted by permission of New Directions Publishing Corporation. Translated by Muriel Rukeyser. U.S. and Canadian rights.

Acknowledgments

The etymological dictionary says that think and thank come from the same root word. Think means a thought, a thank. And so I give this moment of thought, of thank you:

— to you my loved ones — family and friends who have been alive with me, especially through the first edition of the book in 1975 to now

— to you, Irene M. Connelly, my mama Irene friend who inspired me since bringing me into the world

— to you Blaize Connelly-Duggan, Jade Connelly-Duggan, Caeli Connelly-Campbell, Jim Campbell, Bob and Susan Duggan for loving me

— to you my beloved patients

— to you my wonderful students, alumni, teachers, administrators, front desk staff, board members of the Traditional Acupuncture Institute, and the School of Philosophy and Healing in Action (SOPHIA)

— to you, John Wilson, my loving artist

— to you, Elise Hancock, my kindly editor

— to you, Mary Ellen Zorbaugh, my continual inspiration

— to you, Melora Payne, my true friend

— to you, my thoughtful readers for this edition, Nancy Gilfoy, Harwood Beville, Judy Beville, Flor and Jerry Bunker, Marlowe Root, and Kate Goldberg

— to you, Professor J.R. Worsley, my mentor and teacher — the work here is yours seen through my eyes and the charts are all the fruit of your labor

— to you, Ivy Amponsah, and your wonderful children for being my Ghanaian family

— to you Raeford Ellison, Sadie's son, for your tender partnering

— and to you, especially, Katherine Hancock, my wise and noble, compassionate and skillful sidekick.

I place this book in Sadie's memory, and in the memory of Dede and John Levering, my friend Sally's mom and dad. I am continually learning the possibilities of think-thank, which you call me to.

Ch'i Po said: *The utmost in the art of healing can be achieved when there is unity?*

The Emperor inquired: *What is meant by unity*

Ch'i Po answered: *When the minds of the people are closed and wisdom is locked out they remain tied to disease. Yet their feelings and desires should be investigated and made known, their wishes and ideas should be followed; and then it becomes apparent that those who have attained spirit and energy are flourishing and prosperous, while those perish who lose their spirit and energy.*

—A conversation between Ch'i Po, an acupuncture master, and the Yellow Emperor, from the ancient classic *Nei Ching.*

Table of Contents

The movement of the Tao consists in returning...

Tao Te Ching #40

An Update for the 1994 Edition

The main text of this book is not dated. It is based upon nature, and nature continues unrevisable. The elements return, return, return, ever new, ever old, ever present. Winter spring summer late summer fall and over and over again. So, I am not revising. Rather, I am bringing up to date my understandings. It has been twenty years since writing this text: the space of time of twenty cycles of seasons, of experiencing existence, of learning to dance life. I'm reminded of a little story of two girl babies born in the same nursery on the same day. They look over at each other. They are taken home by their families, become toddlers, little girls, become young women, grow older, become older women. Close to the end of life they meet again—look over at each other again. They ask, "Well, what did you learn?"

I am learning more and more to see existence, that is, life itself including death, as a great dance, a dance of simple and profound movements. The poet Stanley Kunitz in his eighty-third cycle of seasons wrote, "gradually, I'm changing to a word" (in the poem "Passing Through"). Though I am only in my forty-ninth cycle of seasons, I begin to think I might know what he means. I begin to see the possibility of the whole of life as an act of love, moment by moment, day by day, season by season simply... just that... embodying the word—love. I am in training, and so are you. I write this as an act of love.

Twenty years ago when I was writing this book, I was 28 and I "could not see to see," as Emily Dickinson says. I did not really *get* the mortality of us all. That we will die and that life is so much about death. Since then I have come to three certainties, and only three:

that we are here alive now;
that we are here together;
and that we will die.

All life is contingency—a kind of awesome happening that interweaves us, that bodies us forth, that "possibles" us from moment to moment until that last unknown point of time. I also did not get the notion of suffering as a serious suchness. Now I am beginning to comprehend that each of us "bears" being alive in a unique circumstance of breath and space. Each is in a dance that we cannot delegate to another, a bearing of the happenings, the occurrences of the day. From these phenomena we get to observe the conclusions we draw, the stories we tell, the interpretations we make. From our pondering upon what life is asking us to bear we construct our unique offerings to each other. We offer from what we suffer. See the root words: *sub* (under) + *ferre* (bear) = *sufferre*; *ob* (toward) + *ferre* (bring) = *offerre*. We bring what we must bear.

In 1975 at the time I was writing this text to complete my PhD, there was very little written in English about acupuncture. Especially there was little about the dance of the five elements and a few folks began to ask for copies. Thus this book's origin was to speak the "Wu Shing," the five movements, to a western world that knew them not; to make a simple offering through which the unity of life could show; from which the beauty and poetry of being alive could enter our daily round.

Now in the world are 80,000 copies plus translations in German and Italian of this work, and letters come from all over to tell me how it has mattered, and still matters to those who are reading it. Over and over again, remembering the simplicity and power of nature, which is the essence of this text, comforts and coaches the one who reads.

Yet there is now so much to read that I have wondered about the ongoing value of this little book. If it is going to continue to be available, dear reader, I wanted to come again to the text to see if it still stands, to see what wants to be added now. And as I look at the case study I wrote 20 years ago, I see how over these 20 years I have come to observe us beings of the human sort with more compassion and humility. In this edition, then, a new case study reflects my deeper knowing that the human being stands between heaven and earth, a bowing servant between the two, arms stretched up toward the heaven and legs down to the earth. The image that we embody the dance is increasingly important to my being a practitioner for life. I have come to see that we are all practitioners for life. We are all in the dance of life, with the universe and with each other. And when we dance most powerfully, we are tending life, life as it occurs through those around us. In the treatment room the unique person there with me is practitioner for those in life with her-him, and the work we do together is for the sake of others. When I ask, "Who beside you will benefit by your being here?" the question recognizes that we are all, as beings of the human sort, here for each other. Each of us, mostly without realizing and claiming it, is practicing the art of being alive.

The more we are wakeful observing that this is so, the more we can give each other the gift of what we are learning, the better we "practice" life.

I began this introduction on the computer (which 20 years ago I did not have) and for days sat stumped by print. No glide of the pen—the "stylo" on the empty page—no "feel" of the paper under my hand—no physical forming of the letters into words. Sacred words of this language holding the worlds of life as I (we?) have come to speak and listen and write them. In script I can get closer—right up close—a kind of natural embodied movement, though as you read this in print, it will not show you what I mean—the longhand of this body writing for you—the letters formed through my unique existence... as you read through the eyes of your unique existence. You also cannot hear my sounds, nor smell my smell, or touch my face, nor I touch you. Even so, through these words we come together—we build a bit more of the world.

Life is not a finished action.
Love is not a completed thought.
Teilhard de Chardin

O me! O life! of the questions of these recurring....
—What good amid these, O me, O life?
    Answer
That you are here—that life exists and identity,
That the powerful play goes on, and you may
contribute a verse.
Walt Whitman
Oh Me! O Life

Dianne M. Connelly
Columbia, Maryland, July 1994

Preface

I have always wanted to be a healer. When I was 10 years old, my father died from a brain tumor that was diagnosed after he was stricken on a bus far away from home. It was then that illness wedged itself into my life like an axe in a tree—and I felt I must seek and dedicate my life to the creation of health. I was a vociferous reader and quite taken in my early teens with Dr. Thomas Dooley—remembering a phrase Dr. Albert Schweitzer once wrote to him: *I do not know what your future will be but this I do know—you will always have happiness if you seek and find how to serve.*

In high school I was in a future physician's club and befriended by a Dr. James Mishkin, who took me on rounds and allowed me to be with him and his patients. I began to understand more and more about disease and its destructive force in people's lives.

In college I studied pre-medical courses, the biological sciences—then in my junior year I went to Rome to an international house. There I took a comparative religions and philosophy seminar, and my head began to turn toward a different way of viewing life, the world and its people; a more composite, less compartmentalized view in which the interconnectedness of life became clearer to me.

I went on—studying philosophy, theology—and got a degree, wondering how to become a healer when each discipline I looked into—biology, psychology, philosophy—seemed to give me bits of life, but none really gave me a focus on the totality of an individual. I studied psychology and anthropology and got an M.A. Still I sought a wholistic look—so far in vain. Western medicine seemed so anatomical—psychology so emotional—I wanted a way of combining everything. Because I needed to earn a living, I took a training program in Montessori and taught two to five years olds in a Bronx Head Start Program. Those little ones taught me more about the life of a human being than any course I had thus far taken. I could see in them a life force and I could hold them in my arms amid shouting, tears, and laughter. Still I felt I had no handle with which to grasp the concepts of health and to use those concepts. I wanted more exposure to life—especially to other ways of thinking and looking.

With my friend Bob Duggan, I went to the Orient to find people who could teach me something about the process of health and human potential. From the Far East and all around the world in what seems now to have been a well-laid path, I arrived at the doorstep of Professor J. R. Worsley in Kenilworth, England. A 10-day stay in a Singapore hospital to find out what the severe abdominal pains and frontal headaches I had were, with no results; rumors of a master acupuncturist in England and a College; my need to find a direction for my life, personal and professional—all brought me to the experience of Traditional Acupuncture.

I was examined and treated. I was, at that time, feeling very low and irritable inside with headaches, menstrual problems and abdominal pain. I was skeptical, much relieved and grateful to be treated as though my complaints were somehow connected and real. After the first treatment I had a moving experience of energy flow, a revitalization of my spirit. But I also had very bad cramps—worse than any previous menstrual ones I had ever had. With some misgiving I went back to Dr. Worsley for my second treatment. He took my pulses and described for me the cramps down to the very time. I could not imagine how he could know such information without my telling him, and until I began to study the diagnostic work of Traditional Acupuncture, I thought he must be a wizard of a man wreaking magic. I was still skeptical and didn't much like the needles (the thought of them was always the worst), but I began to feel so well in myself that I had to admit that something good was happening to me. I was no longer angry and full of pain. In fact, I felt I loved the world. As Dr. Worsley explained more about what he was doing, I realized that I had found what I had been looking for my whole life long—a profession and a way of life that looks at and honors the whole person; a method of healing that does not segment the bodymindspirit: I cried that day.

That was in the autumn. I began my formal studies at the College of Chinese Acupuncture U.K. the following spring, under Professor Worsley.

Dianne M. Connelly

Columbia, Maryland, November 1975

Foreword

Traditional Acupuncture originated in China about 5,000 years ago. It is a complex system of examination, diagnosis and treatment. In its inception it was thought of as preventive medicine, that is, the creation and maintenance of health. We, in the West, have heard most about Acupuncture in its anaesthetic use. This is a relatively recent innovation which explores the relationship between Western surgery and Eastern pain relief. Another form of Acupuncture that we often hear about is known as symptomatic Acupuncture. It is an analgesic first-aid technique that can bring temporary relief from pain without diagnosing the cause. This is also known as the *bare-foot doctor* or formula approach.

Traditional is the form of Acupuncture, that we seldom hear about. There is a great deal of confusion and very little cohesive information written about it. Texts and magazine articles about it tend to be done like cookbooks with the specific ingredients of the recipe but not much talk about the background and experience of the dish itself.

The purpose of this text is to present the healing art of Traditional Acupuncture in depth; to distinguish it from the symptomatic and anaesthetic forms of Acupuncture; to provide a sound conceptual framework from which to view this type of medicine; to explain the process of examination, diagnosis and treatment; to present various case reports. This work is in no sense my creation by the newness of content, but by the synthesis and presentation of it—an Eastern healing art to a Western culture. In writing this I have had to increase my own perceptions.

Traditional Acupuncture is a healing art and science which teaches how to see the entire human being in bodymindspirit, how to recognize the process of health and illness, and how to go about the restoration of lost health in an individual. The main difference between Western medicine and Oriental medicine is the basic theory of the Chinese that there is a Life Force called Ch'i Energy, and that this Life Force flows within us in a harmonious, balanced way. This harmony and balance is health. If the Life Force is not flowing properly, then there is disharmony and imbalance. This is illness.

The usual way that we know we are ill is via a symptom which acts as a signal of distress. This signal tells us that something is wrong. We may feel the distress as a migraine headache, an ulcer, a period of depression, arthritis, insomnia or any other complaint. From the Chinese point of view, these symptoms point to trouble somewhere in the flow of the Ch'i Energy. We could say that the symptom is the trouble in itself and so try to eliminate it, but from the perspective of Traditional Acupuncture, this would be like covering up a flashing generator light in your car when all it's doing is indicating trouble. The problem is not dispelled by disguising the symptom.

A full examination is done using the diagnostic tools of Chinese medicine to assess the condition of the Ch'i Energy and to find the cause of illness. These tools take into consideration everything about a person: for example, the sound of the voice, the hues coming from the face, the predominant emotion, the temperature and texture of the skin, the gait and posture, the childhood history, the favorite tastes, the best and worst times of day, the dreams, the appetite and diet, the ability to sleep, the workings of the bowel and bladder, the sexual energy, the stresses within the family and at work, the acuity of the senses and a person's habits and hobbies. This is not an exhaustive list, but it does give an idea of the range of information that is important in Traditional Acupuncture in order to make an accurate diagnosis of a person's illness. A most important tool in this process is pulse diagnosis.

Each organ is associated with a pulse and other facets of life: an emotion, a taste, a color, a time of day, a season, an odour, a sound, a sense organ, a body orifice, a pathway where the Ch'i Energy flows and so forth. (See correspondences of the Elements in chapters 2–7.) In a very cursory way, this means that a person who has an imbalance in the flow of the Ch'i Energy that controls the kidneys may also be exhibiting related symptoms such as a craving for salt, an excess of fear, a preference for or intense dislike of the color blue, a lack of will power, ear troubles, an abhorrence of cold weather, sexual inadequacy or pains along the specific pathway of Energy that governs the kidneys. Each organ has its correlations. Two people may have the same or similar symptoms, yet the diagnosis and treatment vary extensively.

We continually express what is happening within us. The examination gathers this information and uses it as a basis for diagnosis. A fundamental presumption is that we want to be healthy, that is, to be in harmony and balance within ourselves and within our lives and that the Bodymindspirit will do what it can to make this so. Acupuncture treatment restores order and balance to the Ch'i Energy enabling it to flow clearly without obstruction, so that the Bodymindspirit can then heal itself. Traditional Acupuncture treats the person, not the disease.

The text begins with an introduction to the Five Elements and their correspondences. This is the base of information needed to understand how the Chinese see the relationship of the Elements to health and illness.

Sections of the text discuss each of the Five Elements and the correspondences specific to it: The Elements—Wood, Fire, Earth, Metal, Water; and the correspondences: color, season, organs, time of day, direction, flavor, orifice, sense organ, fluid secretion, emotion, sound of voice, part of body governed, external physical manifestation, power granted, smell, climate—type of weather, storing of a life aspect, dreams, grain, fruit, meat, vegetable, number, musical note, pathways, pulses.

Then follows the section on Examination. This explains and illustrates the procedure of the Traditional Acupuncture examination as it is carried out according to the four basic tenets: to see, to hear, to ask, to feel.

The last section of the main text is on Diagnosis and Treatment. Once the examination is completed and a diagnosis made on the basis of the Five Elements, then treatment is carried out using needles and moxa. This last chapter explains the process of diagnosis and treatment.

In the text there are several concepts about health that fall strange on Western ears; for example: the concepts of Ch'i Energy, YinYang, Bodymindspirit, the Pulses, Five Elements, Meridians, Balance... These are explained at length in the text. They may, at first, require a *willing suspension of disbelief* on the part of the reader because of unfamiliarity. This is not unusual since we, in the West, are only just learning to explore the meanings of health from an Oriental perspective.

This work represents the studies at the College of Chinese Acupuncture U.K. under my mentor Professor J. R. Worsley, Doctor and Master of Traditional Chinese Acupuncture.

As with any work of this nature, I owe a great debt of gratitude to many individuals for sharing ideas and insights, for being patient with me in the process of learning and writing, for editing and typing and re-typing and preparing it for publication. I want to thank all the practitioners associated with The College of Traditional Chinese Acupuncture at Leamington Spa in England and the Acupuncture Clinic at Oxford, England. I especially want to thank my fellow practitioners and excellent staff at The Centre for Traditional Acupuncture at Columbia, Maryland for all their help to me.

I also want to thank all those who come to me for Acupuncture and who constantly teach me so much about the laws of nature.

Section One

Chapter One

Introduction to the Five Elements and Oriental Medicine

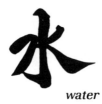

water

fire

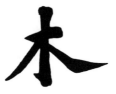

wood

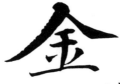

metal

earth

The Five Elements

To the Chinese, and to any people who live from the Earth, the closeness and importance of Nature are understood. They live in the Elements, depend on the cycle of the seasons, survive according to the laws of the universe, and revere the flow and changes of the world around them. They watch, heed, learn and steep themselves in the Elements so basic to life. And, just as Nature all around them is going through its natural process of change, they instinctively know that the Nature inside them follows these same pattens, that intuitively human beings go through the cycle of the seasons within themselves, that the Elements are recreated within them. Each Element is ever present and ever basic to life. It is not just in the world around them that the tender shoots of spring are born bursting into life; it is also within themselves. It is not only in summer that things bloom and flourish, but also within them, and so on with all the seasons. We are the seasons. We are the Elements. Nature is without and within us, each of us every moment. We are a replica of the universe passing from season to season in a natural unending cycle of life.

> *The interaction of the Five Elements brings harmony and everything is in order. At the end of one year the sun has completed its course and everything starts anew with the first season, which is the beginning of Spring. This system is comparable to a ring which has neither beginning or end.*[1]

> *Chinese medical thinking could be expressed, for medicine was but a part of philosophy and religion, both of which propounded oneness with Nature, i.e. the universe.*[2]

All thinking, feeling, and acting are done in accordance with Nature. Chinese medical thinking grew up with the relationship of the human being to Nature in bodymindspirit. And so, the system of examination, diagnosis and treatment is based on natural processes. The concept of health follows laws inherent in Life Energy, inherent in Nature.

Now, when I speak of Energy, I am speaking of the force which we call life. The Chinese term it Ch'i Energy and liken it to the streams, brooks, rivers, lakes, seas, and oceans of Earth. The Life Force flows in us via interconnected pathways. In a way it is like electricity. It flows in a current, and though we can not actually see it, we can see the manifestations of it, and feel the effects of it. In a way it is like the blood flow which, though we usually do not see it, pulses life through us. All life has it, and it converses with every aspect of life. Without this Ch'i Energy, this Life Force, we do not have life, we are dead.

The Chinese saw the existence of humanity and, in fact, all of Nature as dependent upon this Ch'i. It is only by Ch'i that the planets move, the sun shines, the wind blows, the Elements exist. It is only by Ch'i that human beings live and breathe. When Ch'i is flowing all of life's processes are in operation in a rhythmic and harmonious way. This Life Force is the cohesion of our bodymind-spirit, and the integration of the myriad aspects of each individual human being. Ch'i is spoken of with reverence because it is the basis of life and because, if it goes awry, it becomes the basis of disease. Health and illness are defined by this Life Energy. It is this that the Traditional Acupuncturist speaks of balancing if some aspect of this life energy is no longer in harmony with the totality.

Because it is so precious and basic to life, this Vital Force, the Ch'i Energy, asks of every living creature a way of life that preserves it. *Vitality and energy are considered the foundations of life; in order to keep them flourishing they must be protected and the life-giving force must rule.*[3] There is a path to caring for this Life Force on a human level that speaks of balance and harmony. The sages of the ancient classics knew the *secrets* of life because they followed this path. It is called the Way, the Tao. This Tao has been spoken of as the *tranquility at the center of all disturbances.* Life was not an asceticism, for *it aimed at the harmonious function of all the senses, avoiding both deprivation and excess.* There was a *completeness of living, a preservation of the intactness of life.*[4] This intactness touched on all aspects of daily living—food—exercise—thought processes—caring for one's own unity and simplicity—living according to the movement of Nature. One of the people recording the Tao, the Way, is Lao Tzu, whose work is the *Tao Te Ching.* In this book, aphorisms like *A journey of a thousand leagues starts from where your feet stand*[5], and paradoxes like *Keep empty and you will be filled*[6] tell of the spirit of the Tao.

> *The Tao is like an empty bowl,*
> *Which in being used can never be filled up.*
> *Fathomless, it seems to be the origin of all things.*
> *It blunts all sharp edges,*
> *It unties all tangles,*
> *It harmonizes all lights,*
> *It unites the world into one whole.*
> *Hidden in the deeps,*
> *Yet it seems to exist forever.*

I do not know whose child it is;
It seems to be the common ancestor of all, the father of
  things.[7]

These passages give us the sense of life as experienced by the ancient Chinese. Following the Tao was the way of knowing and keeping the Ch'i Energy within them pure and clear, and thus health and happiness could abound.

So, the Ch'i Energy is the vital force in all of life, and the Tao is the Path to sustain the pure Ch'i Energy. The Chinese, then, in watching the universe, saw that this Energy could be spoken of in a dual way, a kind of brother-sister team which they called YinYang. In reality these two are one, but one may be more or less apparent at a certain time. For instance, when night is upon us we do not at that moment experience the day, and yet the day emerges from the night. This we call the dawn, a moment when the YinYang is in nearly perfect balance. When the night emerges from the day, we call this time the dusk, another moment of near perfect balance. We could not know day if not for night, and night if not for day. The world is full of examples of duality which can be called YinYang: for instance, outside-inside are both aspects of something, yet one does not exist without the other; even though we may be looking at the inside of something and not for the moment be seeing the outside, still the two are there simultaneously. All of life has this dual aspect. We usually call them opposites like hot-cold, love-hate, dark-light, active-passive, hard-soft, odd-even, heavy-light, contraction-expansion, sour-sweet, wet-dry, strong-weak, sun-moon, left-right, heaven-earth, masculine-feminine, centripetal-centrifugal.

We tend to think either one or the other of the opposites exists, rather than of both being present with one aspect manifesting more than the other at a given moment. YinYang is not a dialectic of opposites clashing, it is the unity of two aspects of Ch'i Energy whose continual movement revolves in a constant interplay of balance. This interplay moves in a cycle. Neither aspect is more important than the other.

When the Yang has reached its highest point the Yin begins to rise, and when the yin has reached its greatest altitude it begins to decline, and when the moon has waxed to its full it begins to wane. This is the changeless Tao of Heaven. When forces have reached their climax, they begin to weaken and when natural things have become fully agglomerated they begin to disperse. After the year's fullness follows decay, and the keenest joy is followed by sadness. This (too) is the changeless condition of Man.

Liu Tzu of Liu Chou
around +550[8]

Chinese medicine uses YinYang to designate each of the organ systems. For example, the Bladder is considered a yinYANG organ function. It is coupled with the Kidneys, a YINyang organ function. We often hear that something is Yin, or something is Yang. Though this is easier as a system of categorization, it is not correct. There is always some Yin within Yang, some Yang within Yin. One never exists without the other. It is only together that they define the Ch'i Energy.

Though YinYang gives us a facility for working and thinking about vital Ch'i Energy, it is the Five Elements which give us a framework more closely connected with daily life. The Five Elements are Wood, Fire, Earth, Metal, Water. As we look around us at any moment, we can feel the Elements and have a direct experience with them. Essentially this is how the Chinese came to see the importance of Nature. They saw Wood: trees growing, they felt the Fire: the sun, they tilled the Earth beneath their feet, they discovered Metal, they used Water to quench their thirst, they watched the interaction of the Elements as the seasons passed before them. Of the Elements Ch'i Po said, *Their changes, their increasing value, their increasing depreciation serve to give knowledge of death and life...* and the Yellow Emperor said, *In order to bring into harmony the human body one takes as standard the laws of the four seasons and the Five Elements.*[9]

Like YinYang, the Five Elements are further descriptions of the Ch'i Energy as it goes through cyclic transformations. Everything in life is concordant with these Elements, and so not just philosophical and agricultural thought was based on them, but also medical thought. The cause of illness is diagnosed through an examination based on the Law of the Five Elements. Health is the harmonious balanced cyclic interaction of these Elements. Health is maintained only when the Energy flowing through each of the Elements is clear and lifegiving.

The human being is a microcosm of the universe, and so the description of the Energy that activates the cosmos is the same description for the human being. We are YinYang. We are Wood, Fire, Earth, Metal, and Water. Each of our organs is assigned to one of these Elements. Colors, sounds, smells, emotions, time of day, seasons, numbers, flavors, planets, moon phases, powers, form a kaleidoscope with the Elements. The pathways of Energy within our bodies correspond to an Element. As I describe the Elements one at a time, though they are never separate from one another, you will begin to see, as the Chinese saw, how we human beings are a totality. With this vision it becomes clear that the system of

Chinese medicine, and specifically Traditional Acupuncture, is based on a system of correspondences that brings life together for everyone, not just the suffering individual and the student of Chinese medicine. The very core of these correspondences is the Five Elements. To understand them it is necessary to at least be familiar with the concept Bodymindspirit which I have been using throughout.

This concept of Bodymindspirit is the Chinese belief in the unity and integrity of the human person: though there may be different aspects of the self to consider, these aspects can never be isolated from the context of the individual as she is and as she experiences life. The skin is not separate from the emotions, or the emotions separate from the back, or the back separate from the Kidneys, or the Kidneys separate from will and ambition, or will and ambition separate from the Spleen, or the Spleen separate from sexual confidence. I say this because the Chinese make these connections and because it is important to stretch our minds beyond what seems to be disconnected compartments of life, so that we can begin to see the connections and flow of the whole people that we are. The spirit of what I am saying is contained in the following quote:

> My body is in accord with my mind, my mind with my energies, my energies with my spirit, my spirit with Nothing. Whenever the minutest existing thing or the faintest sound affects me, whether it is far away beyond the eight borderlands, or close at hand between my eyebrows and eyelashes, I am bound to know it. However, I do not know whether I perceived it with the seven holes in my head and my four limbs, or knew it through my heart and belly and internal organs...
>
> ... when I had come to the end of everything inside and outside me, my eyes became like my ears, my ears like my nose, my nose like my mouth... My mind concentrated and my body relaxed, bones and flesh fused completely, I did not notice what my body leaned against and my feet trod, I drifted with the wind East and West, like a leaf from a tree or a dry husk, and never know whether it was the wind that rode me or I that rode the wind.

> *Book of Lieh-tzu*[10]

Chinese expression often sounds poetical and allegorical, giving the impression of a beautiful system that smacks of unreality or at least is quite removed from life as we know it. Yet, the system is eminently rational and real. The poetry serves to elucidate the art of the science of Chinese medicine based on the Five Elements. Each Element and its correspondences in human life are as real as the words on this page, as real as the presence of the earth beneath our feet. I say this to make it quite clear that the beauty and common sense of this system of healing in no way detract from its seriousness and depth.

Wood creates Fire, Fire creates Earth, Earth creates Metal, Metal creates Water, Water creates Wood. In Nature we see that Fire is produced by the burning of Wood; Wood is produced by the moisture and rain nourishing it; Metal as a liquid is like Water and as a solid gives the formation of the mountains and beds in which rivulets flow; from the compression and center of the Earth, Metal is produced; from the ashes of Fire and the decomposition created by the sun, Earth is produced; from the forests of the land, Wood is taken to create Fire; from the Water of the Earth, the trees are irrigated and given life; from the Metal of the World come minerals composing Water; from the rocks of the Earth are produced the minerals that make up Metal; from the products of Fire come the lifegiving Earth. On and on the cycle passes from Element to Element in a process of continual creation. Each Element is produced by and produces another. No one of them is more important than another. As I begin to draw out the correlations and meaning of each one, it is important to hold on to this fact that one Element is not more important than another, that, in fact, one does not, and cannot exist without all the others. *The sages combined Water, Fire, Wood, Metal, and Earth ... they held them as inseparable and constant.*[11] This is also true of the functions within each Element because it is there within the Element that we begin to talk about the processes familiar to us like the lungs and breathing, the large intestine and eliminating. So, if we grasp now that each Element and all that it represents is at once supremely important, yet no more important than the next, we start to grasp the significance of the Elements within ourselves. This becomes clear.

Each element has a chapter which provides a description of the Element as it is in Nature along with its correspondences. Each is presented in the following order: The Element—The correspondences:

Color
Season
Organs
Time of Day
Direction
Flavor
Orifice
Sense Organ
Fluid Secretion
Emotion

Sound of Voice
Part of Body Governed
External Physical Manifestation
Power Granted
Smell
Climate—Type of Weather
Storing of a Life Aspect
Dreams
Grain
Fruit
Meat
Vegetable
Number
Musical Note
Pathways
Pulses

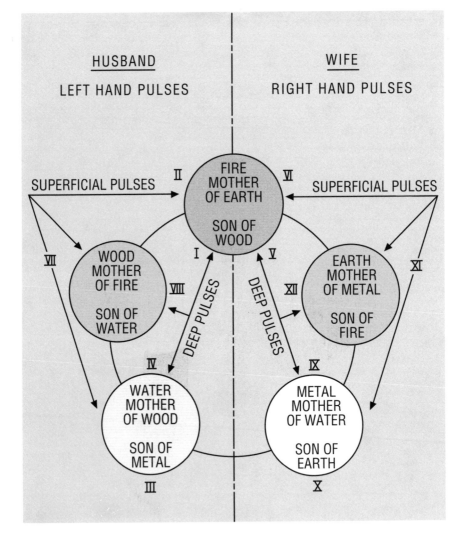

This is adapted with permission from a section of a six-color chart:
The Law of the Five Elements by J.R. Worsley.

© J.R. Worsley, 1972.

Chapter Two

Wood

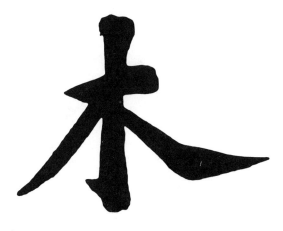

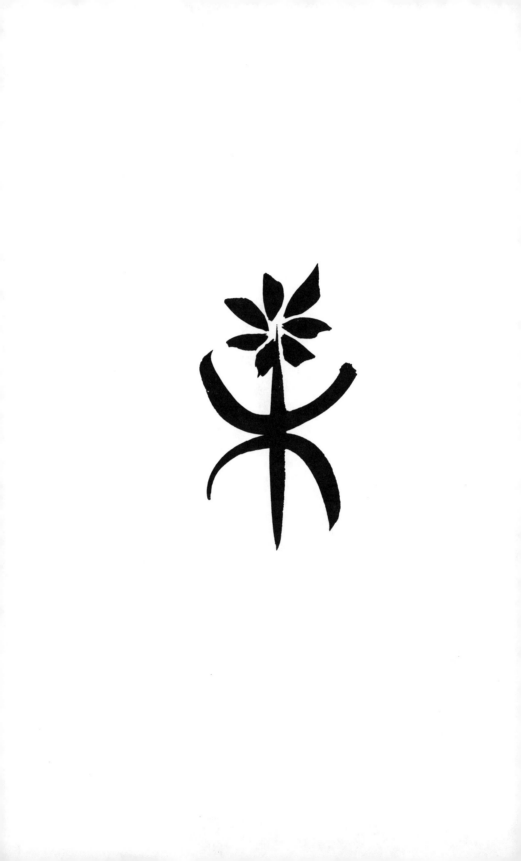

Wood

A pure and simple tree is closest to the concept of Wood. During its life a tree grows. It is a rooted, growing creature reaching out and upward and down and inward simultaneously. It is flexible, bending, yielding to the wind, yet strong and durable, containing the flow of its own life cycle. Beginning from a tiny seed it flourishes as a sapling, its tender shoots heading toward maturity carrying its history with it as it grows, its rings of life. Its connection with the earth and movement toward heaven are witness to the Bodymind-spirit, that is, a composite of the forces of Heaven and Earth within the human being. The tree grows and in growing gives birth again and again to new life. Its cycle marks out the seasons.

We are the Elements; therefore, we are the Element Wood. The description of the tree is also a description of a person. When the human being is flourishing just as the tree in the woods, the Energy, the vital Ch'i Energy is wholesome and clear. The human being is growing and rooted, flexible and strong, carrying the seeds of new life and going through a cycle from season to season. But, what if this is not the description? What if the tree that is the person is not well-rooted and gets pushed over easily? This could manifest itself physically as being off balance and falling over, feeling disconnected with the Earth, being dizzy and uprooted, easily confused, lacking the ability to create roots for one's self, having vertigo. What if the tree has stopped growing? The symptoms that arise could be any type of paralysis, gnarling of limbs (often a description for arthritis), stultification of thoughts and emotions, feelings of smothering, nightmares of being trapped, abdominal pains, cramping. What happens if the tree is planted where it does not get enough nour-ishment or sunlight? The limbs could become weak, or stiff. The trunk would lose its vitality and strength, the vital Energy could not flow. In the human being who is not receiving enough nourishment and sunlight, a similar description could be true, and symptoms would appear to testify to this. Spinal problems may arise if the Element Wood is out of balance, i.e., the *trunk* of the person is in trouble, or there may be problems in the articulation of the limbs, the flexibility of movement, the rootedness of the entire human being. The person who comes to Acupuncture may be coming because her Wood Element needs attention.

The *Color* That Corresponds to Wood is *Green*

There are places on the face where this will show up clearly. If the Ch'i Energy is flowing harmoniously within each Element and among the Elements, the face will not show any predominant color. But if one of the Elements is imbalanced, the color associated with it will show, usually very clearly, on the face. This is not skin color, but rather a subtle hue coming from the face. It is very real and has been used for thousands of years as one of the diagnostic tools in Chinese medicine. *Every disease has a symbol through the variety of the five colors...*[1] *The patient's appearance (color) must be watched high and low, left and right—each where it is most essential.*[2] As we take a look at Nature and see that there the color of the Element Wood is indeed green, especially in the season of Spring, we begin to see for ourselves the correlations the Chinese made. In examination the color green is significant not just in the hue from the face, but also in terms of preference of the patient. If she surrounds herself with green and wears green clothing to the exclusion of other colors, she is pointing to the Wood Element within herself. Also, if she detests green, she may still be pointing to Wood. It is important to remember that an extreme of anything asks us to look at the opposite polarity to begin to see the entire reality. Only then can we start to see balance.

The *Season* That Corresponds to Wood is *Spring*

Planting and begetting are in accord with spring...[3] *The three months of 'Spring' are called the period of the beginning and development (of life). The breaths of Heaven and Earth are prepared to give birth; thus everything is developing and flourishing.*[4] *Everything is restored at the beginning of Spring.*[5] *Spring is the time of the beginning of the creation of all living beings; therefore their breath is still flowing softly and weakly, their pulse is slow and slippery, but they keep themselves upright and straight and are in the process of growing, and therefore one compares them to the strings of a lute. When the condition is opposite then they are sick.*[6] Spring is the time for birth and in the ancient tradition, as you can see from the excerpts from the *Nei Ching*, the springtime gives the power to the world, the Element Wood and the human being to come alive, to be infused with the vital Ch'i Energy, to grow, to be reborn. There are people who are ill who feel that everything inside of them is dead, finished. There is no spark, no interest in life, no coming alive, no being born again. The spring within them is asking to be created or they will die. Some people will say that their ailments are worse in the spring than at any other time, or that spring is the only time that they feel good. The Bodymindspirit tells us to look at Nature as the pattern of the human person so that from Nature we can diagnose and treat. In the season of spring we do literally sow the seeds for the fall harvest within ourselves. The Traditional Acupuncturist knows that unless the seeds of healing are sown in their proper season through treatment, the tree—that is the person—will not thrive.

The *Organs* Associated With the Element Wood are the *Liver* and *Gall Bladder*

When we speak about organs, it is essential to note that the Chinese think about the organs as functions operating on all levels of the bodymind. . . . *the liver has the functions of a military leader who excels in his strategic planning; the gall bladder occupies the position of an important and upright official who excels through his decisions and judgement. . .*[7] Thus, an organ like the Liver takes on a wider and seemingly less scientific meaning than the Western mind ordinarily gives it. The function of planning takes place everywhere in the human being, and, for that matter, in the universe. The flow of the Energy within us happens according to plan. When that planning stops or falters for any reason, symptoms arise which indicate that is happening. For example, a migraine headache may show itself when the Energy of the Liver is in trouble, a sort of frustration within the system because plans were not laid out or being followed. A person with an imbalance in the Element Wood, of which the Liver is a part, may describe a migraine as a *jamming up in the head so that I can't think, or plan, or do anything.* This is only one of several symptoms that could arise from lack of planning.

The sister organ to the Liver is the Gall Bladder whose function of decision making works closely with planning. I imagine we have all known someone who has difficulty making decisions, real difficulty to the point of impossibility even on little things. It is not unlikely that this inability points to an imbalance in the Gall Bladder functioning. Decision making is happening continuously within our bodyminds. Anything that goes wrong with that process will show itself as symptoms related somewhere in the system of correspondences in the Wood Element.

The *Time of Day* Associated With the Wood Element

There is a natural law called the Law of Midday-Midnight, the Body Clock. It provides a daily chronology for the Five Elements, that is, a time when each of the organs within the Element is functioning at its *peak* of energy. For the Gall Bladder this time is *11:00 P.M. to 1:00 A.M.* and for the Liver it is *1:00 A.M. to 3:00 A.M.* During the traditional examination, one of the questions asked is whether or not there is a time when the patient feels better or worse during the day. One person with a Wood imbalance could not sleep at night until 3:00 A.M. During this time his thinking was absolutely clear. He spent the late night-early morning hours doing legal reports for the next day because it was the only time he felt good enough to do them. Often, if a pain is connected with the Gall Bladder or Liver, it will ease during the hours that the Element Wood is at its *peak.*

> *Ch'i Po answered: The East creates the wind; wind creates wood; wood creates the sour flavor; the sour flavor strengthens the liver; the liver nourishes the muscles; the muscles strengthen the heart; and the liver governs the eyes. The eyes see the darkness and mystery of Heaven and they discover Tao, the Right Way, among mankind.*

> *The supernatural (powers) create wind in Heaven and they create wood upon earth. Within the body they create muscles and of the five viscera they create the liver. Of the colors they create the green color and of the musical notes they create the note 'chio'; and they give to the human voice the ability to form a shouting sound. In times of excitement and change they grant the capacity for control. Of the orifices they create the eyes, of the flavors they create the sour flavor, and of the emotions they create anger.*[8]

> *Yellow Emperor's Classic*
> *of Internal Medicine*

This excerpt summarizes the correspondences of the Wood Element. A Traditional Acupuncturist finds these vital in diagnosis.

The *Direction* Associated With Wood is *East*

Beginning and creation come from the East.[9] There are certain diseases that are said to correlate to the East. The wind that relates to Wood is an East wind which can be injurious to the Liver. An elderly patient with painful arthritic hips told me one day that the only thing that he knew that could make the pain worse was an East wind. Without realizing the Chinese tradition, he had pointed to his imbalance in Wood.

For Wood the *Taste* is *Sour*

It is frequently found that a person who loves vinegary kinds of things is feeding a Wood imbalance, or trying to right it. This is an example of the bodymind's natural sense of what it needs, even though we might never have been able to verbalize why we have a craving for a particular taste. According to the classics, the flavors affect our functioning. *If people pay attention to the five flavors and blend them well, their bones will remain straight, their muscles will remain tender and young, breath and blood will circulate freely, the pores will be in fine texture, and consequently breath and bones will be filled with the essence of life.*[10] Each of the flavors has an effect on the Energy, and so the combination of the five insures balance. An excess of any one of the flavors has an injurious effect, and yet, each Element can be strengthened if the right flavor is prescribed for it. *When the heart suffers from tardiness, one should quickly eat sour (food) which has an astringent effect.*[11] *One uses pungent food in connection with the Liver in order to supplement its function and to stop leaks, and one uses sour food in order to drain and expel.*[12] *The excess of sour flavor toughens the flesh.*[13] *If too much sour flavor is used in food, the flesh hardens and wrinkles and the lips become slack.*[14] The association of sour with Wood is referred to by J. Needham in *Science and Civilization in China,* Vol. II.: *wood, as vegetal, would be connected with all kinds of plant substances which became sour on decomposition.*[15] As far as I can gather, every correspondence has had a basis somewhere in daily life, a kind of organic growth process over 5,000 years providing a base for Acupuncture diagnosis and treatment.

The *Eyes* Are The *Orifice* of Wood

When the liver receives the blood it strengthens the vision.[16] In any eye problem one would look to the functions within Wood, that is, the Liver and Gall Bladder, to see if the Energy there has lost its clarity and balance. When we consider that the functions of these two are those of decision making, judgement and planning, it makes sense that the organ of vision is connected with them. Even on the simplest level it takes vision and *sight* to make plans and decide.

The *Eyes* Are The *Sense Organ* of Wood

The eyes are the sense organ as well as the orifice for the Wood Element. In conjunction with this, the fluid secretion connected with Wood is tears, the *water flowing from the eyes . . . in regard to the liver the secretions become tears.*[17] The *eyes* are considered to be vessels of vision integrating the outside and the inside of a human being. When we *see* we take into ourselves information which we use as a guide for what we do, and how we think. The eyes, governed by Wood, need to be clear and unencumbered in order to be used to see. *The eye must be brilliant of perception. . .*[18] Blindness, dimness of vision, astigmatism, short and long sightedness, cataracts, pain in the eyes, distorted vision of any sort, any symptoms of the eyes are governed by the Wood Element and therefore in some way related to the balance of Energy in the Liver and Gall Bladder. It is not difficult to see the value of this knowledge in making a diagnosis.

The *Emotion* Corresponding to Wood is *Anger*

A person with an imbalance in Wood will have a marked presence of anger in themselves, or a complete absence of anger. An excess of anger is injurious to the Liver and Gall Bladder. An excess could mean a feeling of being *stuck* there as though paralysed, unable to escape anger whatever the experience. It could mean feeling irritable continually, and *on edge* with others; always wanting to pick a fight with someone; angry with one's self for no apparent reasons. On the other hand, there could be an inability to express anger or feelings of frustration and inner conflict. The healthy state of the human being is to be able to feel and express all of the five emotions and their variations as it is appropriate. Every illness, that is, every imbalance of the Energy is bound up with an emotion.

The *Sound* Corresponding to Wood is *Shouting*

This makes immediate sense considering the emotion of anger associated with Wood. It is usually a subtle pervasive tone in a person's voice, but oftentimes this particular sound is blatant. Whatever a person says is a kind of shout, aggressive and forceful, continuously. It is important to remember that this sound is a symptom, a cry for help as clear and as real as a broken arm.

The *Parts of the Body* Governed by Wood are the *Muscles and Sinews*

. . . the liver harbors the force of life of the muscles and the thin membranes.[19] The statement refers to tendons and ligaments more than muscles. Muscles are what give us our physical strength or, if they are not in shape, give us our weakness; but the tendons and ligaments hold us together—they bind us physically so that we have mobility. Diseases affecting the tendons are most often attributed to the state of the Ch'i energy in the Wood Element. Fatigue of any sort is thought to also be connected with Wood, *The liver causes utmost weariness . . . and is effective upon the muscles. . .*[20]

The *External Physical* Manifestations of Wood are the *Nails, Hands and Feet*

The condition of the finger and toe nails shows when the liver is in a splendid and flourishing condition. . .[21] Since nails are so visible, people often notice changes in their nails before any other symptoms appear. The variety of change—e.g., striation, coloring, splitting, peeling, cracking, ridging—tells something about the energy in the Wood Element. Each of the Elements has some external manifestation.

The *Power* Granted by Wood is the *Capacity for Control*[22]

This correlates rather obviously to the functions of planning, judgement and decision making of the Liver and Gall Bladder and to the correspondence of the muscles and tendons, which most certainly speak about the power of control within our bodies. Lack of coordination, feelings of panic and desperation, weakness can be symptoms of this human power going askew.

The *Smell* Associated with Wood is *Rancid*

In the classic *Nei Ching* this smell is also described as *offensive and fetid.*[23] In another source it is described as *urine or sour sweet.*[24] It is very difficult to actually give a word for the peculiarity of this odour, but there is a definite association of it with an imbalance in Wood. The character for the smell in Chinese seems to defy an exact translation into English.

The *Climate* Connected with Wood is *Wind*

. . . the wind circulates within the liver. . .[25] *The east wind arises in Spring; its sickness is located in the liver and there are disturbances in the throat and neck.*[26] *If the wind enters the body and exhausts man's breath, then his essence will be lost and the evil influences will injure his liver.*[27] *. . . wind is the cause of a hundred diseases.*[28] The Chinese believed the wind to be a potent force in the lives of human beings, so potent it could do injury to the Ch'i energy. It is one of the external forces which, when experienced in excess, that i⸍ prolonged exposed contact, can result in illness. A patient's clim⸍ preference in the traditional diagnosis is based on the assoc⸍ of climate with Energy.

The *Life Aspect* Stored in Wood is the *Spiritual F*

The liver is the dwelling place of the soul. . .[29] *The live⸍ soul and the spiritual faculties. . .*[30] In a way this is or⸍

difficult of the correspondences to understand because it makes us ask questions about what is the soul, the spirit and what they mean to us, as well as what they meant to the Chinese in terms of diagnosis. *Once the spirit has turned away it will—as a rule—not return.*[31]

The Emperor asked: *And what is meant by shen, the spirit?*

Ch'i Po answered: *Let me discuss shen, the spirit. What is the spirit? The spirit cannot be heard with the ear. The eye must be brilliant of perception and the heart must be open and attentive, and then the spirit is suddenly revealed through one's own consciousness. It cannot be expressed through the mouth; only the heart can express all that can be looked upon.*

I think it is important to remember that because the Chinese did not dichotomize the individual, their base for talking about the spirit was integral to the whole human being. Acupuncture was a method for curing illness, and illness resided in the entirety of the person including the spirit. In fact, *the spirit of a person was the first aspect considered necessary to cure,* and only then the other aspects of the individual could be cured.

The method of the needle (acupuncture) is available to all people. The first method cures the spirit; the second gives knowledge of how to nourish the body. . . In order to make all acupuncture thorough and effective one must first cure the spirit.[33]

A person whose desire for life is gone, or a person whose life style puts excess stress on the bodymind, is not following what the Chinese considered central to life. It is most difficult to help someone who does not want to get well, that is, does not have the spirit. The same is true for those whose lives feed the imbalances of the Energy within them. Taking care of one's self, keeping the balance, nourishing the Bodymindspirit is part of the process of staying healthy. When we come to a discussion of acupuncture points we find that each point has a spirit, an essential dynamic which can bring about change within the Energy.

Dreams Associated with and Corresponding to Wood

A question regarding dreams and nightmares is asked during the Acupuncture examination. Information from them correlates with what is happening with the Energy. In *The Theoretical Foundations of Chinese Medicine*, Porkert talks about dream motifs which indicate malfunctions of the Liver and Gall Bladder. If the energy in Wood is *exhausted, in dreaming one will see mushrooms; at the right moment one has the sensation of lying under a tree and not daring 'o get up.* If the Energy is deficient *one dreams of trees in a mountain 'rest. . .*[34] *one dreams that one is engaged in fights and battles or that one cuts open one's own body.*[35] Certain paradigms occur in dreams that tell the state of the YinYang balance, as well as information about the patient's view of herself. There are dream therapies today which use the information from dreams in a way similar to the ancient Chinese method of diagnosis. Dreams often give a handle to the physician and patient about the course of illness. They are not used as the sole tool for diagnosis, but together with information of all the correspondences within an Element.

The *Other* Correspondences

The correspondences given so far are the major ones used in Chinese medicine. There are several others. For example, every Element has a grain related to it. *The five grains act as nourishment.*[36] For Wood, the grain is *wheat.* Every Element has a fruit. *The five fruits from the trees serve to augment.* For Wood the fruit is the *peach.* Every Element has a domestic animal which gives additional nourishment. For Wood the meat is *chicken or fowl.* There is a vegetable for each Element. It is said to finish the nourishment for that Element. For Wood the vegetable is the *mallow.* These . . . *unite and conform to each other in order to supply the beneficial essence (of life).*[37] The combination of these with the foods corresponding to all the other Elements is considered to be a sound, harmonious and healthy diet.

There is a number associated with each Element. It is said to be the number of the order of completion of the Element as it was evolved from heaven and earth. The number for the Wood Element is *eight.* Obscurity surrounds the actual usage of these numbers in Chinese medicine. Though a person with a major imbalance in the Element Wood might have a special affinity or aversion for the number eight, it is probably stretching it a bit to anticipate that this will be so.

Musical notes are also ascribed to each of the Elements. There are five that come from the old pentatonic scale. The (sound) musical note for Wood is *chio.* The tone of this is said to be likened to the lute. The sound of the lute is said to be the description of the Energy flowing through the Wood pulses. *In Spring (the season of Wood) the pulse is like the strings of a lute. . .*[38]

The *Pathways*

The Ch'i Energy flowing in the Element Wood has two major pathways (also called Meridians), along which the Energy flows and can be altered. The first pathway correlates to the *Liver* and is located on the body beginning at the big toe, running up along the front inside of the leg, onto the torso and ending there just at the lower edge of the thoracic cage.

Though the pathway goes to a deeper level, at that point we speak of it as *ending* since only along the described meridian are there points where the Acupuncture needles can effect changes in the Energy. There are 14 points on this meridian and they are bilateral. In the examination we feel the Energy along this pathway to know if it is blocked, especially if a patient is complaining of something which seems related to the Element Wood and in particular the Liver Meridian.

The second pathway in the Wood Element correlates to the *Gall Bladder*. It is along this Meridian that a needle can be inserted to effect a change in the Energy and functioning of the Gall Bladder. This pathway begins by the side of the eye, runs along the top of the ear then back up along the head twice, then down along the neck to the front of the body, down the outside of the leg to the foot, ending at the fourth toe on the side toward the little toe. This pathway has 44 points, that is, 44 places bilaterally where a needle can be inserted to bring about a change in the Energy of the organ system of the Gall Bladder. Knowing where this pathway travels, we can see that symptoms of the eyes, ears, head, torso, legs and feet all could be connected with an Energy imbalance in the Gall Bladder Meridians.

It is not only the anatomical organ, the Gall Bladder, that is affected by an imbalance of Energy in this pathway. With each anatomical organ, the Energy that relates to it travels a pathway that affects other parts of the bodymind as much as it does the structure of the organ itself. So we find problems with the eyes connected to the Gall Bladder and Liver, hence one of the reasons for the correspondence of the eyes to the Element Wood (see *Orifice* and *Sense Organ*). The location of the pathways is also important for the patient to know since there is often a sensation that moves in one direction or another once the needle is inserted into a point along the pathway. The description of this sensation can often guide the Traditional Acupuncturist in assessing the Energy as it enters or leaves the pathway.

The *Pulses*

The last and greatest correspondence of the Element Wood is that of the two pulses used as the diagnostic gauge for the state of the Energy within the Element. A reminder is needed here that we are the Elements and that what is going on with us reflects the Energy flow within us. In order to be able to discern this Energy flow, all of the above correspondences are considered. The pulses give us the most exact and best reading of the Energy. (For description of pulse taking see *To Feel.*) In a way all the other information is a footnote to the pulses, a verification that what is being found is true.

> *... the feeling of the pulse is the most important medium of diagnosis. Nothing surpasses the examination of the pulse, for with it errors cannot be committed.*[39]

The pulses are the reading of the state of Energy in the bodymind. Each of the other correspondences tells us either a little bit about the Energy or what Element to look at as the one being most in need of balancing, but it is the pulses which focus all this information.

The pulse for the Liver and Gall Bladder are read on the left hand. The position of the finger (the 2nd position) is the same for both, but the depth of palpation is different. The pressure is slightly stronger for the deeper pulse, which is the Liver. Within the pulse is all the information of the Bodymindspirit. The Traditional Acupuncturist spends her whole life developing this skill to the exquisite sensitivity needed to be able to discern the past, present and future imbalances. Life, the Chinese believed, and its description are there in the pulses for those humble and clever enough to feel.

Chapter Three

Fire

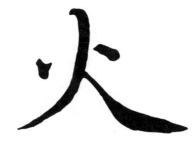

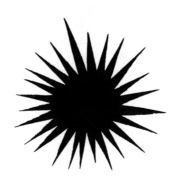

Fire

What is the Element Fire? It is warmth and light, and it creates warmth and light. It is dynamic and moving, full of spark, vitality; brilliant in its activity, lively and colorful. To come into contact with it is to feel its presence. It can be used for creating Energy and to direct it. To be *on fire* is to be full of excitement about life. To be *all fired up* is to be propelled by enthusiasm about something. Fire always refers to life in some way. It is a life principle. Fire is active, it rises up. Its essence is alive. A spark, a flame, a blaze give us images of what Fire is. A Fire in the homely hearth creates the atmosphere of warmth and love. The sun is Fire, its rhythm in our lives, its symbolism as life giver, its reality as part of the life cycle, its warming, nourishing rays. We are Fire.

Let me take just one of the concepts associated with Fire and apply it to us human beings, that is, the concept of being warm and giving warmth. The healthy human being needs warmth, is warm and can give warmth to others. But what of the person who is not healthy, who has no Fire inside and so is cold physically and emotionally. There are so many symptoms the bodymind may use to express trouble in the Element Fire: hot painful joints which act as though Fire has lodged in certain places, and is raging there; fevers; feeling parched and arid in mind, body and spirit; lack of emotional warmth and receptivity to other human beings, even those who are close; sexual coldness because the Fire has gone out, and cannot be rekindled; poor circulation of the blood experienced as cold extremities, varicose veins, hemorrhoids, hot flushes; heartburn and digestive problems.

As with the Element Wood, the Fire Element has the same categories of correspondences, but these are the correspondences specific to Fire. They give us information in order to diagnose the state of the Ch'i Energy in the Bodymindspirit as it relates to Fire.

The *Color* Associated with Fire is *Red*

An imbalance in this Element will show on the face as a red hue. *When their color is red like blood they are without life.*[1] However, the complete absence of red, a sort of ashen color may also be a sign of imbalance in Fire. Loving or detesting red points to imbalance within Fire. *The appearance and complexion must be watched high and low, to the left and to the right, for each has its significance.*[2]

The *Season* That Corresponds to Fire is *Summer*

It is said that *the three months of Summer are called the period of luxurious growth. The breaths of Heaven and Earth intermingle and are beneficial. Everything is in bloom and begins to bear fruit. The summer is the time for the protection of one's development.*[3] *In Summer, the pulse is that of the heart; and Fire is the Element of the South. All things in creation flourish and grow, therefore, the breath of all living creatures is plentiful in coming, and decreases in leaving, and thus it is said to be like a hammer. When the condition is the opposite, then they are sick.*[4] What happens in Nature in the summer also happens in the human being; blossoms yield to fruit in the process of ripening, things come to fruition, the Earth is full of plenty, life and warmth. The Chinese considered the same process of fruition, ripening, to be happening with thought, experience, the body and emotions. Seeds are sown in the spring. Seedlings grow until they blossom, housing tiny fruits which grow and, when ready, fall to the earth. What happens if there is no bloom and the fruit does not grow, but withers and loses its life? The symptoms of this within a person could be not being able to finish anything one starts; losing feeling and the capacity for use of a limb; a general malaise in which nothing gets done. From inside the sick person, the resemblance to what happens in Nature outside her is very real and provides a handle to understand her own processes. *A sickness particular to the middle part of Summer is located within the chest and ribs.*[5]

The *Organs* Associated With the Element Fire are the *Heart* and the *Small Intestines*

Along with these are two functions called Circulation Sex and Three Heater.

The heart is like the minister of the monarch who excels through insight and understanding. The heart fills the role of 'sovereign ruler' from whom emanate directing influence and clear insight.[6] Professor Worsley describes it as the Supreme Controller overseeing the workings of the bodymindspirit.[7] In Acupuncture writings the Japanese deem the Heart to be sacred, and so rarely treat it directly. Imagine what happens when the monarch becomes ill and there is chaos in the domain of the bodymind, a kind of inner panic and loss of control. The internal peace and harmony shake and a person experiences symptoms proclaiming the tenuous state.

The small intestines are like the officials who are trusted with riches, and create changes of the physical substance.[8] According to Porkert the Small Intestine has the role of the *organ that receives and assimilates the bulk of food. In other terms, in it the fine and the crude, the clear and the murky elements of food are separated and redistributed.* Professor Worsley describes it as *The Separator of Pure from Impure.* This happens on all levels of our experience. There is always this sorting out process going on, the keeping of nutritional value and passing on the waste to where it can be removed from the bodymind. We can rightfully say that there is a small intestine of the emotions, the ideas, the thoughts; a sorting out of rubbish from essentials. If this sorting out function is not operating in top form, the symptoms that arise express the confusion of the bodymind. An example of this might be hearing difficulties, which could be described as the inability to sort out sounds from each other, or digestion problems, which are the result of poor sorting. In a Western context one could not readily imagine the Small Intestines having anything to do with the ears. Imagine what happens within the other functions of the bodymind, for example with the *decision maker*, the gall bladder, if the sorter is not doing her proper work. Decisions are difficult and frustrating with unclear information. It is little wonder we feel it when something goes wrong with one of our vital functions. We can also begin to see the scope of each function as we realize the areas of life they relate to.

Though the function of *Circulation Sex* does not have an organ structure, it is often thought to be associated with the pericardium, the muscle of the heart. The *Nei Ching* says that Circulation Sex, *the middle of the thorax (the part between the breasts), is like the official of the center who guides the subjects in their joys and pleasures.*[9] Manfred Porkert translates it to be an *official ambassador.* Professor Worsley speaks of Circulation Sex as the *Protector of the Heart.* It is in charge of blood flow and sexual secretions. As Protector, it guards the functions of the Supreme Controller so that her work carries on uninterruptedly. The Protector takes the bumps, bruises and traumas which the Controller would receive if it were not being protected. Circulation Sex is like a buffer taking hard blows so that the integrity of the bodymind stays intact. Imagine how weary and worn out she gets if the day, the months, the years have been full of heavy blows. Imagine if those blows had pounded on the Heart itself.

Because of her close relationship with the Heart, Circulation Sex can also be characterised by the association we make with the Heart. For example, love relationships of any and all sorts are guarded by this function; the vitality and nourishment of blood flowing through our vessels is controlled by it; the lubrication facilitating ease and flow in sexual experience depends on it. The pulse of life is governed by Circulation Sex. We can well imagine what happens if the Energy within Circulation Sex is not in harmony with itself or the rest of the bodymindspirit. It wields tremendous power and balance. Hundreds of symptoms attributable to this function go mistakenly diagnosed or undiagnosed in Western medicine just because this function is unrecognized. The recognition of Circulation Sex along with the Three Heater is perhaps the greatest gift traditional Chinese medicine has to offer the Western world of therapies and the ailments of sick people.

The *Three Heater,* also called Triple Warmer or Triple Heater, is the sister function of Circulation Sex, and thus works closely with it. Though there is no anatomical organ correlative to the Three Heater, the Chinese believe that all of the organs in the body are guarded by it and that heat is controlled by this function. There are specific references in the *Nei Ching* to the *burning spaces* and their relationship to the Lungs, and the waterways of the Bladder and Kidneys. *The three burning spaces are like the officials who plan the construction of ditches and sluices and they create waterways.*[10] *The atmosphere of their lungs will be blocked from the lower burning space.*[11] The three burning spaces are known as the Three Chou.

The Three Chou divide the torso of the body into three areas. *One examines by feeling with the hand the three sections of the body . . . as to whether they are overly abundant or wanting, and one brings them into harmony.*[12] Each space corresponds to certain internal organs. For example, the Heart and the Lungs correspond to the Upper Chou (burning space); the Stomach, Spleen, Gall Bladder, Liver and Small Intestine correspond to the Middle Chou; the Large Intestines, Bladder and Kidneys correspond to the Lower Chou. From these correspondences we see the connection of the Three Heater with respiration, digestion and elimination.

The Three Heater is the heating system of the bodymindspirit. It maintains temperature and warmth at optimum conditions for the whole system to carry on its daily chores in comfort, harmony and balance. All Three Chou must be in harmony with one another in order for each one to coordinate the temperature of the oxygen systems within its jurisdiction. If this function were out of balance, all of the warmth of the bodymind could go askew causing hot and cold emotional and physical upsets like a kind of yoyo within the system.

Because the Three Heater corresponds to all the organs, whenever something goes wrong with the energy of any one of the organs one might first go to the Three Heater to see how strong and clear that

Energy is. Unless the Three Heater is considered with all the other functions, one cannot correctly diagnose the cause of a person's illness. Circulation Sex and Three Heater are two of our most powerful functions. All relationships depend on them for harmony, warmth and connection.

The *Time* Associated with Fire

There are two times of day for Fire. The Heart is at its peak time between 11:00 A.M. and 1:00 P.M., followed by the Small Intestines from 1:00 to 3:00 P.M. Then, at 7:00 P.M. to 9:00 P.M. is the time of Circulation Sex, followed by the Three Heater at 9:00 P.M. to 11:00 P.M. These are based on sun time. If we lived in the rhythm and cycle of the sun, all of our natural functions would take their order. A good example of this sun cycle is the timing for the two Fire functions, Circulation Sex (7–9 P.M.) and Three Heater (9–11 P.M.). The natural time to be in bed, and thus the natural time for making love, is just after the sun goes down, which is no doubt why Circulation Sex and Three Heater are associated with those hours.

> *From the South there comes extreme heat. Heat produces fire and fire produces the bitter flavor. The bitter flavor strengthens the heart, the heart nourishes the blood and the blood enlivens the stomach. The heart rules over the tongue.*
>
> *The (supernatural) powers of Summer create heat in Heaven and fire upon Earth. They create the pulse within the body and the heat within the viscera. Of the colors they create the red color and of the musical notes they create 'chih' and they give the human voice the ability to express joy. In times of excitement and change they grant the capacity for sadness and grief. Of the orifices they create the mouth with its palate; of the flavors they create the bitter flavor, and of the emotions they create happiness and joy.*[13]

The above excerpt gives a brief description of the other correspondences with Fire. The language of the classics is often a bit obscure, but the essence is clear, and it is the essence of the correlations which serves as the basis for diagnosis.

The *Direction* for Fire is *South*

Nourishment and growth come from the South.[14] Certain diseases are said to correlate with the South according to the *Nei Ching. Their diseases are bent and contracted muscles and numbness....*[15] Apparently the predominance of these symptoms occurred in the South, giving rise to this correspondence. The center unbilical pulse points to the Fire Element if it is off in the direction of the South.

The *Flavor* Corresponding to Fire is *Bitter*

If too much bitter flavor is used in food, the skin becomes withered and the body hair falls out. The heart craves the bitter flavor.[16] *The bitter flavor has a strengthening effect.*[17] A description of bitter with Fire is given by Joseph Needham: *The association of bitterness with Fire, while perhaps the least obvious of the five, may imply the use of heat in preparing decoctions of medicinal plants, which would be the bitterest substances likely to be known. There would also be a connection of 'hot' and bitter in spices.*[18] The taste of bitter is difficult to find compared to sweet, but things like green leafy vegetables, coffee, tea, chocolate (without sugar), anything charcoaled or burned, are bitter. This flavor has to be integrated into a person's diet to balance out the other tastes. An imbalance in the Fire Element would likely give rise to an extreme regarding the bitter flavor.

The *Ears* Are the *Orifice* of Fire

Red is the color of the South, it pervades the heart and lays open the ears. . . .[19] We have spoken of the Small Intestines as part of the Fire Element and the connection with the functioning of the ears, as they sort out sounds. Ear aches, ringing, deafness of all variations, hearing anamolies are all linked with the functions of Fire. This means that the Heart as *Supreme Controller*, the Small Intestines as *Separator of Pure from Impure*, Circulation Sex as the *Protector of the Heart* and Three Heater as *Warmth and Maintenance Official* are all involved in the process of hearing as it relates to the ears. In the pathways correspondence you see that the Meridians of Fire are located near the ears.

The *Tongue* is the *Sense Organ* of Fire

The mouth with its palate[20] There is a difference between this and the mouth itself which relates to the Earth Element and to the Metal Element. The tongue's appearance provides information about the Fire Element, especially about the Heart and the circulation. This information is also known in a Western medical context. Even though the tongue generically describes Fire, it is also divided into segments which give information about each of the Elements. *The heart rules over the tongue.*[21] Because speech is largely controlled by the tongue, many speech patterns and impediments like stuttering and slurring may be symptoms of a Fire imbalance. Via speech we express who we are to the world around us, and by hearing we discover through sound who the world around us is. Both of these senses which presume relationship are based in the Element most governing relationship, that is, Fire. It should *not* be concluded that because something is governed by one Element that the other Elements are excluded from that facet of life. The Elements are so intimately bound up with one another they can never really be separated or isolated one from the other.

Perspiration is the *Fluid Secretion* of Fire

. . .*it leaks out through the pores of the skin.*[22] Sweat is an interesting natural phenomenon often taken for granted. The Chinese recognized its place in the preservation of life, and were aware of the consequences, a lack of or overabundance of perspiration might mean to the human being's proper functioning. . . .*if people do not perspire freely in the heat of summer, they will get intermittent fever in fall. If people perspire (only) partially, they contract a partial paralysis. When perspiration becomes visible and meets with humidity, there will be eruptions on the skin and a weakened condition.*[24] For some diseases it was thought that if perspiration could be brought about, the disease would be broken and terminated. This is a familiar concept in the Western world concerning certain types of fevers. The Chinese believed perspiration to be an *unclogging*[25] allowing the bodymind to be cleansed throughout. Though perspiration is most often associated with Fire, this secretion is a good example of the interconnection of the Elements since overexertion within any Element may create variables of perspiration.

After heavy eating and drinking perspiration is produced by the stomach. When man is shocked and startled he does violence to his spirit and vitality, and perspiration is produced by the heart. When man carries a heavy burden while taking a long journey, perspiration is produced by the kidneys. When man, during rapid marching, is apprehensive and full of fear, perspiration is produced by the liver. When the body is shaken in hard toil perspiration is produced by the spleen.[26]

I think it is well to note at this point the concept of uniqueness inherent in the Chinese view of the person. Because two people may express the same symptom does not mean that their diagnosis and treatments would be identical. In fact, this is the reason Traditional Chinese Acupuncture does not diagnose via symptoms. Symptomatic Acupuncture runs the risk of misdiagnosis by not viewing the person as a whole, and so missing the distinct, unique cry for help.

Joy and Happiness are the *Emotions* of Fire

Poets for eons have associated the Heart with happiness and sadness. *Broken hearts, half-heartedness, goodheartedness, faint* hearted, lion hearted. . . .describe a human condition in basic simple language. As well as referring to joy, they also refer to the psychic strength surrounding the Element Fire, of which the Heart is a function. The Protector of the Heart, Circulation Sex, has also to do with the preservation of joy, the balance of pleasure in our lives. The ancient sages lived so that . . . *in their pleasures and joys they were dignified and tranquil. They followed their own desires and they never directed their will and ambition toward the protection of a purpose that was empty of meaning.*[27] The Chinese in their wisdom concerning balance realized that the emotion of joy in excess is as harmful as an excess of anger; the lack of joy is just as harmful. The desire for permanent joy is an impossible thirst and, if sought after inordinately through work or play, can put too much stress on the Fire Element, causing something to *give.* Often the symptom of high blood pressure is the bodymind's way of saying, *Take it easy or I'll succumb to this pressure.* Heart attacks are often the final straw, a desperate attempt of the bodymind to alert us to the excessive striving, hence the actual deficiency of the emotion joy. Within this stress there is often a great deal of sexual frustration. An imbalance in the emotion of Fire almost always revolves around relationship in a person's life.

The *Sound* Corresponding to Fire is *Laughing*

This is a subtle, though sometimes blatantly obvious, sound in a person's voice no matter what the person is saying. A hint of laughter often pervades even the saddest conversation of a person with a Fire imbalance; a sound that is oftentimes a continuous giggle, irrepressible and evasive. Often the complete absence of laughter accompanies a Fire imbalance. Either extreme is significant. A never-ending jokester is the other side of the serious, humorless, joyless person.

The *Parts of the Body* Governed by Fire are the *Blood Vessels*

The Fire Element governs the Blood Vessels of the body and therefore the pulse of all the organs. *The viscera are in thorough communication and bound by circulation with the heart, and the blood that is stored by the heart, and thus the blood fills the pulse with the force of life (breath).*[28] This means that the flow and circulation of blood, which nourishes all the rest of the body, are controlled by the Element Fire. Therefore, as we might expect, such labels as hardening of the arteries, varicose veins, cold hands and feet, thrombosis are all symptoms arising from an imbalance in Fire.

The *External Physical* Manifestation of Fire is the *Complexion*

The complexion of a person shows when the heart is in a splendid condition.[29] A Traditional Acupuncture practitioner looks at a person's face closely to see what is happening there because it serves as such a strong guide to the Fire Element. This is not the same as the colors emanating from the face; it is more a description of the face texture, quality, and skin.

The *Power* Granted by Fire is the *Capacity for Sadness and Grief*

This is a power bestowed upon every person. It relates to joy and happiness as the balance in human life, since the human condition demands that we learn to accept and give witness to things that call for sadness. This capacity is spoken of *in times of excitement and change,*[30] which are the times when meeting and parting, the old and the new, are present to each other. At these moments the ultimacy and poignancy of human life are felt deeply, a kind of *peak* experience, a moment of consciousness.

The *Smell* Associated with Fire is *Scorched*

Any major imbalance in Fire can be smelled on a person's body. It is unmistakable once experienced, and in some cases overpowering. This is not the body odour, but rather a distinct other scent. Considering that it is the Element Fire, it makes empirical sense that the smell would be a scorched, burnt odour.

The *Climate* Connected with Fire is *Heat*

Heat is injurious to the heart.[31] Corresponding to this is the south wind, which is said to cause the *ailments of the heart, chest and ribs.* An excess of hot weather can upset the balance within Fire, and thus affect any or all of the four functions already discussed. Heat is an external force to be contended with so that it does not injure the bodymind. A person who abhors hot or even warm weather, or loves it, cannot thrive without it, is likely to be expressing an imbalance of Fire. *When the elements of heart conflict (within the body), they cause sudden pains at the heart, hidden troubles, dangerous vomiting, headaches, red complexion, and lack of perspiration.*[32]

The *Life Aspect* Controlled by Fire is the *Spirit*[33]

Of the Heart, which is one of the representatives of the Fire Element, the Classics say it *is the root of life and causes the versatility of the spiritual faculties.*[34] *... the heart stores and harbors the divine spirit.*[35] This is the terminology of the ancient Chinese, and though it may not be acceptable as they phrased it to our Western ears, the principles they suggest are familiar and essential to life. Inherent in the human being is a yearning for health defined by the Chinese as harmony and balance among the Elements within us. This yearning has a dynamism one could call spirit, a principle of consciousness providing a milieu for experience, a vital centre from which to live. Imagine if this yearning, this spirit, begins to dissipate. The integrity of the human experience crumbles too, creating confusion, desperation, joylessness. There is no heart left, and so all the vital forces break down. That is how important the spirit is to the ill person in whom the desire for harmony is waning. Here is where the criminal, disgusted and violent with life, is crying out for help.

The *Dreams* Corresponding to Fire are Nearly Predictable

An imbalance in Fire produces dreams where one is *looking for fire...*, *at the right moments one (even) dreams of fire and blazes.*[36] This is when the Heart is exhausted. Porkert also translates: when the Heart is full of abundant energy *one easily laughs in dreams or is afraid.* In an acute deficiency of Energy *in one's dreams there appear hills and mountains or blazing flames.*[37] (Translated by Porkert from the classic *Ling Shu.*) If the dream motif is *of populous town districts and of main thoroughfares*, then this is indicative of an acute deficiency in the Small Intestines. Dreams offer evidence of the workings of our Energy even when we are not conscious of its workings within us. As an aid to diagnosis, they are used to verify and explore elemental imbalances.

The *Other* Correspondences

Associated with Fire is the grain *glutinous millet;* the fruit, the *plum;* the meat is *mutton*, or *lamb;* the vegetable is *coarse greens.* All of these combined with the food associations of the other Elements are the basis of a healthy and nourishing diet. Knowledge of food correspondences is used in treatment. The number associated with Fire is *seven.* This is derived from the philosophy of the origin of the Elements. Earth engendered Fire and Heaven completed it seventh in the order of generation and completion.

The musical note associated with the Fire Element is *chih*. It is likened to the sound of the thirty-six-reed mouth organ. The note is derived from the pentatonic scale. *One must understand that music consists of five notes,*[38] *the five viscera are connected with the five musical notes which can be discerned and recognized.*[39] The viscera are considered the YINyang organs; that is, the Heart, the Liver, the Kidneys, the Lungs, and the Spleen.

The *Pathways*

These correspond to the Heart, Small Intestines, Circulation Sex and Three Heater. Along these pathways (meridians) are the Acupuncture points from which the energy within Fire can be restored to balance. These Meridians are essential to know in great detail when it comes to treatment, so that no mistakes occur either in location of points, the spirit of points, or the overall view of the Energy flow in the external and internal pathway associated with each organ.

I hesitate to keep mentioning the organs and their functions by the Western labels. To the Chinese, the Heart, as an example, meant much more than the anatomical structure associated with it. The pathways corresponding to the organs belong to the sphere of the organ whose scope is integral to the whole human system. It is misleading to say that there is a problem in the Heart without realizing that what the Chinese meant by Heart and its sphere of influence is not the same as what the Westerner means.

The pathway of the Heart begins under the armpit, at the base of the axilla. It travels up the arm and ends at a point near the inside of the nail on the little finger. The meridian is bilateral and has nine points, all very powerful for moving the energy corresponding to the sphere of the Heart. By the sound of the names of the points like *Spirit Path* and *Spirit Gate*, we begin to sense the workings of the Energy in this Meridian. Like all the other pathways, the Heart Meridian goes to a deeper level and connects at junctions with the other functions and so affects the Energy flow there. Though it is true that no one function in the body is *the* most important, the Heart as the *Supreme Controller* is treated with great reverence, and never taken for granted. In fact, in Japanese Acupuncture texts, one gets the impression that the Heart was too sacred to be touched.

One day in class, while learning to locate the points of the Heart Meridian, a student was told to be more gentle in his palpation so as not to influence the Energy in the pathway. It was too late. Blood rushed to his face making it beet red, and he fainted. Professor Worsley had to revive him with the use of other Acupuncture points.

The pathway of the Small Intestines, the sister Meridian of the Heart, begins at the nail on the outside of the little finger bilaterally. It travels up the arm, along the back of the shoulder on the scapula, up along the neck onto the face, where it ends with the 19th point in front of the ear. This point is called *Listening Palace*, giving us a clue to the spirit of the point and the pathway, thus making the connection between the Small Intestines and the ears more apparent.

The pathway of Circulation Sex begins in the fourth intercostal space (between the ribs) just lateral to the nipple. It is bilateral and travels down the arm, across the inside of the hand, ending with the ninth point at the nail on the inside of the middle finger. From the discussion of the function of Circulation Sex it is not surprising to find names like *Heavenly Pond, Heavenly Spring, Palace of Weariness*, suggesting the spirit of Circulation Sex, one of the functions of the Fire Element.

The pathway of the Three Heater, the sister Meridian of Circulation Sex, begins at the nail on the outside of the middle ring finger, travels up along the arm on the outside, over the shoulder, up along the neck, under and behind the ear and ends at the side of the eyebrow. The meridian is bilateral and has twenty-three points. Names like *Pure Cold Abyss, Secretion Gate, Meeting Ancestors* bring us to explore the Three Heater Meridian more closely. The Three Heater is said to be concerned with *balance of sympathies and antipathies, warming family relationships and social ties, and accompanying rupture of relations, estrangements, despair, deep depression, suspicions, anxieties and agitation.*

The *Pulse*

The pulse correspondences for the Element Fire are those used for gauging the state of the Ch'i Energy of the four functions within the Element. *One must first ascertain the pulses...; then one can define the intervening time, and at last one can establish the dates of life and death.*[40] *The pulse of the Heart should sound like the blows of a hammer (continuous).*[41] *To treat and to cure disease means to examine ... the pulse, as to whether it is flourishing or deteriorating, and whether the disease is a recent one.*[42]

The Emperor asked: *What will happen when there is an excess of pulse action in Summer? Will the disease then affect the entire system?*

Ch'i Po answered: *Excess causes man's body to be hot and his skin and flesh to ache; his body will gradually be flooded and unable to live, he will have heart trouble; coughing and spitting will make their appearance above, while below the breath of life is caused to leak out.*[43]

There are many descriptions of the pulses in the ancient classics. I quote several because they speak clearly for themselves of the meaning of the pulse in Chinese medicine. The following quote describes the pulses as they relate to preventative Acupuncture: *The pulse has ways of indicating whether the patient follows or disobeys the laws of the four seasons and whether or not there are hidden symptoms...* The following is a description of the Heart pulse:

When man is serene and healthy the pulse of the heart flows and connects, just as pearls are joined together or like a string of red jade—then one can speak of a healthy heart.

When man is sick the pulse of his heart rushes and pants. When this panting is continuous and springs from within and the pulse beats are wrong and small—then one can speak of a sick heart.

At the point of death the pulse of the heart flows in front but is faulty and feeble in back, and then it stands still as if restrained by a belt or hook—and then one can speak of the death of the heart.[44]

Those who wish to know the inner body feel the pulse and have thus the fundamentals for diagnosis.[45]

It must be remembered that the pulses we are speaking about are specific Energy pulses and not the blood flow pulse, even though the Energy pulses are located along arterial paths, especially easy to feel over the radial artery on the wrists.

The pulses for the Heart and Small Intestines are read on the left hand in the first position. The superficial pressure finds the Small Intestines pulse, the deeper pressure finds the Heart pulse. The palpation is gentle and done with great concentration, quiet and clarity.

The pulses for Circulation Sex and Three Heater are read on the right hand in the third position. The superficial pressure finds the Three Heater pulse, the deeper pressure finds the Circulation Sex pulse. Each of the pulses has a sister, which is why two are read in the same position though at different pressure. These are the couples. The pulses read in the superficial position are yinYANG, and the pulses read in the deep position are YINyang. This is important since this coupling maintains the balance of the two inseparable cosmic forces already discussed, and upon which the Ch'i Energy depends for balance, that is, YinYang.

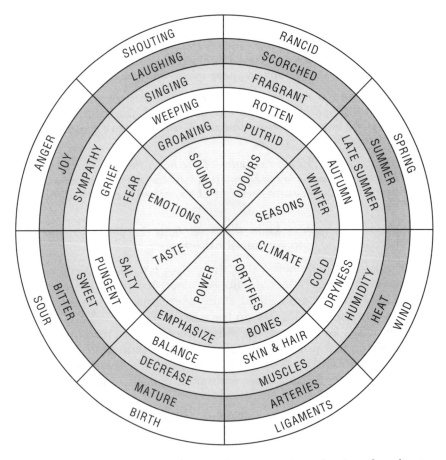

This is adapted with permission from a section of a six-color chart:
The Law of the Five Elements by J.R. Worsley.

© J.R. Worsley, 1972.

Chapter Four

Earth

Earth

What is the Element Earth? It is the ground beneath our feet, the connection we have with the world in which we live and the entire universe. Mother Earth she has been called, from whom we get nourishment, support, life. The foods we eat are grown from the Earth. The place where our feet stand this very moment is on the Earth. The solidarity of who we are is determined by how we posit ourselves in this life on Earth. Fertility, fecundity, fullness are associated with Earth. Stability, basic-ness, essentiality are associated with Earth. To be *earthy* is to bear a certain aura of life rooted deep in the essence of sensuality. The earth is round; therefore, all roundness, contours, circles, and cycles signify the earth. She rotates on her own axis always following a circular path. Cycles of life are within her jurisdiction. Earth is special among all the Elements, because she is the source of them, the centre from which they arise. Each of the Elements is in constant relationship with her, coming to life and dying within her realm; for example, in Wood, the tree is centered and grows within and out of the Earth. Works have been written describing Earth as both womb and tomb, the beginning and the ending, the never-ending cycle of life and death, rebirth. The phoenix rises from the ashes, yearly reborn, from the Earth. The roots of our very being are in the Earth and it is from there that we feed. Being *grounded* is an existential experience of who we are in relationship to the Earth, that is, balanced and stable among the forces of the world ... forces that are physical, psychological, and spiritual. Equanimity and equilibrium stem from our connection with the Earth. Being connected, feeling ourselves to be an integral part of the life within and around us has to do with the Earth. Having a centre from which we operate, a kind of order and harmony emanating from within, rather than chaotic desperate energy, is a description of Earth within us. Being at home with one's self, integrated, unobsessed and at ease wherever we are is a description of Earth. We are balanced and centered within, interacting and connected without.

From this description it is possible to imagine the person whose Earth is sick. All the things I have mentioned may begin to go crazy like cycles losing their patterns. This will occur not just in the most obvious rhythms of life, like the menstrual flow, but all kinds of rhythms like sleeping, breathing, thought processing, body harmony and coordination. Named diseases like ulcers, anorexia (loss of appetite), indigestion, obesity, vomiting, abdominal edema (swelling), hyperacidity and epigastric pain spasms must in some way be speaking to us about the Earth Element. In fact, whatever has to do with the intake of nourishment and the process of getting nourished must be connected with this Element. Other labeled problems like amenorrhea, menorrhagia, dysmenorrhea—all of which have to do with the menstrual cycle—speak of the interruption of a natural flow, a rhythm out of the natural harmony, which most surely speaks of Earth imbalance. The person suffering due to an Earth imbalance may have symptoms of equilibrium, equanimity, grounding gone awry. Nervousness, flightiness, instability, loss of balance, feeling *unearthed,* disconnected, alone, homeless are signs of distress in the Earth Element. Not feeling secure in one's self and depending on the presence of someone else as a measure of existence may be a cry of help from Earth. The egocentric label on the person who claims *I* as everything is asking for someone to pay attention to her Earth and help her find her own ground and center. Many weight problems come from bad distribution of energy in the Earth Element.

The person who has difficulty with sterility may be saying *my Earth is not fertile enough,* and often problems with conception and birth occur when the Element Earth has not been prepared and nourished properly. Seeds planted in arid soil that is not attended and encouraged will not take root and grow, or if they do, may have a hard time coming to fruition. And it is likely that the fruit they bear will be scrawny and nutritionally deprived as well. The milieu of the human seeds must be rich and balanced and well-tended to if the life that begins to grow is to thrive and to bear the journey of life as a healthy balanced being. Within this discussion is one of the meanings, carried in traditional Chinese medicine, of preventative medicine. If we care for ourselves by creating health, the children to whom we give birth must then be healthy and strong in life, learning to create harmony in the same way. The concept of preventative medicine is really that of emphasizing the creation of health.

The *Color* Associated with Earth is *Yellow*

As I have already mentioned in regard to the previous Elements, the color given in association with each Element is a very significant part of traditional Chinese diagnosis. The subtle hue of yellow emanating from the face of a person who is ill tells us the condition of Earth within that person. In speaking of illness and the color of a person, the *Nei Ching* says ... *when their color is yellow like that of oranges they are without life.*[1] This means that the color betrays the gravity of the illness, the imbalance within Earth.

Late Summer, Often Called Indian Summer, is the *Season* of Earth

This is not properly a season, yet experientially Indian summer is truly a specific and separate time of the year. It feels like a combination of spring and summer, to me, with a hint of the autumn about to happen and a suggestion of hidden winter ... a time of great poignancy as though the clock has stopped and all the Elements of life are simultaneously present. In fact, in some of the old texts, this season was said to be the last ten days of each of the four seasons, and so a combination of them all. In the insect world, more furious activity goes on during this period of late summer than at any other time of the year. There is a tremendous metamorphic change within a short period of clock time, a kind of time distortion. The forces of Nature are very precisely balanced and interacting every moment. The same is true in the human being. The Indian Summer of our bodymindspirit is in the midst of great changes taking place within. It is a time when the connection with the Earth is very important to an individual so that the changes do not throw a person into chaos and confusion.

The *Direction* of the Earth is *Center*

Everything that is created by the Universe meets in the center and is absorbed by the Earth.[2] This is not surprising in the light of what Earth the Element is for us. It is central. To the ancient Chinese the two forces Heaven and Earth are responsible for engineering and completing Nature, and all of its aspects. Earth is central to our human creation. In terms of health, if we have no center we have no place from which to balance and order our lives. It is also significant that the pulse at the umbilicus is examined to make sure it is on center during the traditional examination.

The *Organs* Associated with the Element Earth are the *Spleen* and the *Stomach*

The Spleen is also talked of as a Spleen-Pancreas in some texts, but since to the Chinese it means so much more than just the anatomical structure, we use the word Spleen on its own to indicate this function. In the *Nei Ching* the Spleen is considered the source of life for other organs. It is said that the *five viscera all desire their breath of life from the Spleen; it is the Spleen that is the foundation of existence of the five viscera.*[3] In another place the Spleen is talked of as distributing secretions. Dr. Worsley speaks of the Spleen as the *Official in Charge of Distribution*, the *Transporter of Energy*. He likens this transportation system to the best of our modern systems of distribution to and from all parts of the globe. If this Official were not on her toes every moment, parts of the bodymind would not receive the energy they need. The symptoms of this might be a *deadness* of feeling, malcoordination throughout the system, lack of proper sexual transport like spermatorrhea, itching or starvation of some part of the bodymind, or inundation. All of these may tell us that the Spleen is imbalanced, and cannot carry on her proper functioning. *The Spleen is an essential factor and it creates the connection. The Spleen corresponds to the Earth. It regulates the center...* From it everything is carried out to the rest of the body-mind domain, that is, to the four corners of the Earth.

The Stomach's function according to the *Nei Ching* is to act as *the Official of the Public Granaries and grant the five tastes.*[4] And, in another place: *The stomach acts as a place of accumulation for water and grain and as a source of supply for the six bowels.*[5] *... Thus all force of life and all the flavors go towards the stomach where they are digested...* Dr. Worsley speaks of the Stomach as the *Official of Rotting and Ripening*, that is, the one who receives nourishment, integrates it and brings it to fruition, and passes on the food energy to be distributed by the Spleen. In every season, the life-giving force of the Stomach is just as essential to the well-being of the individual. In fact, the Stomach comes close to being *the* most important function in our bodymind because from it our energy feeds, and all aspects of life are taken in. From food the *Rotter and Ripener* culls the essential nourishment and readies it to pass on for distribution. If this function is sick, whatever is taken in, whether it be food for our somatic growth or food for our psychic growth, will not benefit us because it will not be correctly utilized by the bodymind. Energy will not be derived from food if this function collapses. Energy depletion will quickly ensue. Lethargy, weakness and debilitation may be symptoms telling us that the energy is low due to the condition of the Element Earth in the cycle of the Five Elements. Many digestion problems are connected with an Earth imbalance, particularly the function of the *Rotter and Ripener* meridian, that is, the Stomach. The phrase *I cannot stomach this* is not an idle one. It means I cannot take it in, something is unpalatable about it or I am just incapable of assimilating it.

The *Time of Day* for the Stomach is *7:00 to 9:00 A.M.* and for the Spleen *9:00 to 11:00 A.M.*

During these times the energy within Earth reaches a peak. This can be thought of in a commonsense way. Breakfast is considered to be the most important meal of the day. That is when we can best take in nourishment and digest it. This is usually done in the morning in most working households before 9:00 A.M., which is the time of the Stomach. Once the food starts the process of digestion, the process of distribution follows. This is the function of the Spleen whose time follows immediately.

The *Flavor* Corresponding to Earth is *Sweet*

There are many people who crave sweets and would say without a moment's hesitation when asked, *What is your favorite taste? Oh, I just adore sweet things.* There are some obvious commonsense relationships here. The Spleen-Pancreas is the function known in Western medicine to be concerned with named diseases like diabetes, hypoglycemia, hyperglycemia, all of which have to do with sugar in the body. The Spleen is a function of the Earth Element, which is correlated with the taste of sweet in Chinese medicine. This is not to say that the diseases named are the only ones connected with this Element, or that a person who craves sweets must, therefore, be suffering from one of these diseases. The flavors are a clue, and are not in themselves the cause of imbalance. They guide us to look especially carefully at one Element or another. It is also possible that a person who intensely dislikes sweets is providing as valuable a clue to the imbalanced Element as an intense taste preference provides. Joseph Needham describes the association of sweet with Earth as *due to the finding of honey in bees' nests in the earth, and to the general sweet taste of cereals.*[6]

Each of the flavors has a specific effect on the Energy. A balance of them gives a harmonious diet, too much of one flavor can be injurious. The *Nei Ching* says, for example, that *if too much sweet flavor is used in food the bones ache and the hair on the head falls out.*[7] The Stomach is thought of as the dispenser of the five tastes, the storehouse of all the flavors, even though it is part of the Element Earth whose specific flavor is sweet.

The *Mouth* is the *Orifice* Governed by the Earth Element

Our food nourishment comes into our bodies through our mouths. In early development children focus on the mouth. We breathe through the mouth, and breath is nourishment. Food and drink and air are the fuels of our being, the sustenance for the Life Force. This is the main reason why we should breathe, drink and eat pure, unpolluted air, fluids and foods. This is an important facet of health, that is, the taking in of good nourishment via balanced eating, drinking and breathing, which gets vastly overlooked in the maintenance of health. What comes into us via our mouths becomes us in the process of assimilation. There are a number of illnesses aggravated by poor diet and breathing habits and lack of proper nourishment. Many diseases related to the mouth are due to some imbalance within Earth. In fact, the lips often clearly show the state of the Energy within the Stomach and Spleen, the two functions of Earth. The throat is also associated with the mouth orifice.

The *Fluid Secretion* Corresponding to the Earth Element is *Saliva*

This is a close correspondence with the orifice of the mouth. Whenever a person complains of a lack of, or excess of, saliva the Element Earth should be attended to first. Also swallowing difficulties usually point to Earth. If the secretions of the mouth are not flowing properly, then the digestion of the food cannot be done properly without extra strain on the entire digestive process.

The *External Physical* Manifestation of the Earth Element is the *Flesh*

The flesh refers to the covering of the body, the musculature which gives shape to each human being. *The spleen harbors the force of life of the flesh.*[8] The tone, texture, and temperature of the flesh are diagnostic clues to the state of the energy. This is not the same as the skin or the muscles with which we mechanically move. Porkert calls this the *somatic element.*[9] The word *fleshy* gives a description of the concept of flesh. People who have pains in their flesh can often be very specific, knowing that they do not have pains in their bones, joints or muscles. Illnesses that pertain to the wasting away of flesh are often due to an Earth imbalance. The flesh shows whether there is lack of nutrition in a person. Is the flesh slack, firm, taut, tight, or flabby? The description of it reflects the state of the Earth Energy.

The *Emotion* Corresponding to Earth is *Sympathy*

This is also thought of as compassion. As with all emotions, a person who is healthy in bodymind flows from one emotion to another, including that of sympathy. The person who cannot receive sympathy, and the person who asks for sympathy continually, are both *stuck* and do not flow easily in and out of the emotion. This shows in attitude, posture, words and actions. You may not think there is such a thing as too much compassion, and it is often easier to note when there is compassion lacking, but there are people who obsessively look for sympathy from everyone, even to the point of manufacturing complaints in order to find it, and there are also those who sympathize with others to the point of being obsequious. This is not a natural flow and points to an imbalance in the Earth Element. The *I need. . .*, the craving sympathy says that the Earth is imbalanced in the same way someone craving sweets is signalling an Earth imbalance. Health is a balance of needs and emotions.

The *Sound* Corresponding to the Element Earth is *Singing*

This does not mean that all singers have an Earth imbalance! What it does mean is that some people sing whenever they speak. It is usually a subtle, but nonetheless distinct sound. Sometimes it is melodious, sometimes sing-song or monotone, regardless of the words a person is using. This singing sound points to an imbalance of Earth.

The *Power* Granted by Earth is the *Capacity for Belching*

This is also translated as the capacity for obstinancy, which can range from obsession of sticking to an idea, to the strength in sticking to one's guns in the face of odds. When we consider that belching is part of the process of taking in food and the digestion of it, the capacity to belch makes sense when connected to the Stomach, as the process of rotting and ripening occurs. An excess of belching points to an Earth imbalance.

The *Smell* Associated with Earth is *Fragrant*

It is the sort of fragrance, however, that is not pleasant in the usual sense of fragrant. It is a cloying, sickening-sweet smell when it is the smell of an Earth malfunction. The smells are very difficult to describe in words unless one has had the experience of them directly. They are then unmistakable. This particular odour is akin to the smell of flesh burning. (This is not uncommon in countries like Bali where corpses are burned over an open fire in public.) It is not the scorch, but the sweetness that is most overwhelming.

The *Climate* Associated with Earth is *Dampness* or *Humidity*

An excess of dampness can injure the functions of the Earth Element. Weather has always affected the lives of human beings, sometimes beneficially, oftentimes disruptively. People living in a particular climate adjust to it. If they were to go into a different climate, they would experience a physical and emotional trauma. For example, someone from a tropical setting visiting a cold wintery climate would likely suffer some imbalance due to the change. The body can make adjustments rather well as long as the conditions are not extreme. Excess humidity can imbalance the energy in Earth. A person who can stand no humidity or a person who loves humidity is giving information related to the state of the energy in Earth.

The *Life Aspect* for Earth is Associated with *Ideas* and *Opinions*

Within this association are thoughts, inspirations, insights, a connection with one's own views and thought processes. Also included here are obsessions, dogmas, the opinions that become inflexible, the ideas that seem to wither instead of flourish. All of these relate to the Energy of Earth. Intractability, extreme dogmatism, pugnacious tenacity to a certain idea, the inability to conclude thoughts or create ideas point to an imbalance in Earth.

The *Dreams* Corresponding to Earth

Dreams corresponding to Earth can be that of a lack of food and drink, of putting up buildings or walls, of chanting and playing music, of a heavy body and difficulty in rising, of the appearance of hills and marshes, of ruined buildings, and storms.[10]

The *Other* Correspondences

Associated with Earth is the grain *millet,* the fruit *apricot,* the meat *beef,* the vegetable *scallions.* All of these in combination with the other Elements will provide a nourishing diet. These correspondences are not exhaustive but do provide a basic guide to balanced eating. Each person must choose what combination of food is best for the growth and maintenance of health.

The number associated with Earth is *five.* Five is the number of its generation from Heaven according to the tradition of the theory of creation. Heaven and Earth work together for the creation of the Elements, which number five altogether.

The *Musical Note* Associated with Earth

The musical note associated with Earth is *kung,* or the sound of the drum. According to the ancient classics the sounds of music are manifestations of energy, and that music is an expression of harmony and balance of the Elements.

The *Pathways*

The Ch'i Energy flowing in Earth has two major pathways. These correspond to the Stomach and Spleen, which we have discussed in terms of function. The pathway of the Stomach begins on the face under the eye and runs down along the front of the body bilaterally parallel to the center line of the body, then continues down along the outside of the legs and ends at the second toe, on the side of the nail toward the third toe. It has 45 points, making it the second largest Meridian of the body. From the description of the pathway, you can see that points along it cover the full length of the body. This makes it easier to understand why the Chinese think of the Stomach as more than the anatomical structure in the abdomen. There are points on this pathway with names like *Abundant Reservoir, Ch'i Rushing, Heavenly Pivot, Lubrication Food Gate,* giving the spirit of the Stomach and describing its functioning in the entirety of the bodymind.

The pathway of the Spleen begins on the big toe, travels up the inside of the leg and up the front of the body, ending on the rib cage in the sixth intercostal space. The spirit of this Meridian is expressed in the names of the points, like *Earth Motivator, Great Commander of Junctions, Heavenly Stream, Abdomen Sorrow, Encircling Glory.* There are twenty-one points on the Spleen Meridian. Each of them can be used to alter the Energy within the pathway. In the discussion of treatment (see last chapter), I will talk about how points are chosen in order to effect specific changes in the energy.

The *pulses* for the Earth Element are read on the right hand in the second position. The Stomach is read at the superficial level, and the Spleen is read at the deeper level in the same position. According to the *Nei Ching* the pulse of the Stomach and Spleen is very specifically discussed, and like all the pulses is read by the volume and quality of the energy passing through them. *In Summer the pulse of the Stomach should be like the beats of a fine hammer; then it is healthy and well-balanced.*[11] This is one example of description regarding pulses. Each pulse is read separately, but all form a cohesive, harmonious picture of the whole person.

Chapter Five

Metal

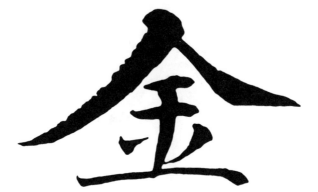

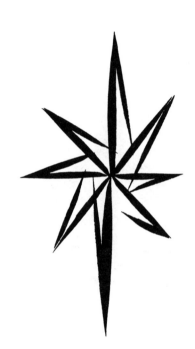

Metal

This is often the most difficult Element to experience in nature. The usual concepts of Metal tend to give the impression of it as cold and hard and not life-giving or nourishing in any human way. It is important to see the part that Metal plays in nature and in us since it describes us as much as the other Elements do.

Who are we as the Element Metal? The minerals of the earth provide substance and richness to the soil from which food is grown. The *salt* of the earth suggests the essence of Metal. Ores are Metal. They are the intensity of the earth. Some provide fuel for heat, others material for structural strength, others—gems for beauty. Consider what a jewel is, the crystalline clarity of its beauty and its symbolic meaning of endurance, longlasting, life preservation, and love all give a feeling for the nature of Metal. I like to concentrate on the aspect of the Metal Element which is associated with substance, strength, and structure. Most structures we have in some way rely on Metal for reinforcement, bolstering, and uprightness. Metal provides a main ingredient in systems of communication. You cannot imagine the world of telephoning, televising, telegraphing, and transportation without dependence on Metal. Metal gives us a substance with which to build networks. Wires connect all sorts of things, holding them together, helping them to function. Metal conducts electricity. Consider mountain streams and rivulets. The pathways in which they flow are a network formed by the Metal of the Earth. If we think of the vast network of the human body, the structure of being able to take in food and air, to assimilate and utilize the fuel, then to let go of the unnecessary things, these are some life-sustaining aspects of the Element Metal. From this description of the Element we could anticipate the signals that would let us know there is an imbalance. For example, problems with structure itself and the strength within the bodymind are often symptoms of Metal imbalance. Symptoms like rheumatic pains, degeneration or rigidity of the vertebral column, specific kinds of headaches, trembling, spasms of the throat, the oesophagus, the limbs, certain kinds of paralysis, debilitating diseases, lack of emotional strength, and incoherent speech might occur. The person whose energy is imbalanced in Metal needs help in rebuilding the network within the bodymind which keeps all the processes communicating. A breakdown in communication can cause dissension, rebellion and disintegration of necessary structure within the entire individual. When I write about the specific functions of Metal—the Lungs and Large Intestine—I will describe what that breakdown can mean.

The *Color* Associated with the Element Metal is *White*

An imbalance of energy within Metal will show on a person's face. It is not the skin color, but rather a hue coming from the face. The *Nei Ching* describes the white in relation to health: *When their color is white like dried and withered bones they are without life.*[1] The color white showing from the face can tell the experienced eye how ill a person is and whether or not she will get better. Diagnostically the association of white with the Element Metal is also used by finding a patient's preference in color.

The *Season* Associated with Metal is *Autumn*

Autumn is the time of harvesting, a reaping of the fruits of the rest of the year, a time to prepare for protection from the winter. *The three months of Fall are called the period of tranquility of one's conduct ... Soul and spirit should be gathered together in order to make the breath of Fall tranquil ... all of this is the method for the protection of one's harvest.*[2] In the autumn *all things in creation approach their harvest, perfection and completion.*[3] Autumn in New England brandishes the changes of that season. Leaves turn vibrant colors, signifying the point of a cycle wherein all things begin to conserve and store themselves inside for nourishment, while externally life seems to be fading. The *autumn of our lives* is a phrase used to give the same feeling of change as do the leaves growing colorful and beginning to fall to the earth. There is often an acute awareness of time passing and growing old in autumn. For some people autumn is a time of transition and sadness, sometimes of desperation and an effort to grab hold of the past and stop the passage of time if only for a moment. One is reminded of Keats' *Ode on a Grecian Urn*, figures captured in activity for all eternity. Autumn is a time for pulling together all of one's resources, for harvesting.

As this is true in Nature, it is also true within each of us, a kind of harvesting takes place with our own energies. Consolidation and strengths as well as fragmentation and weaknesses become clear. What happens if a person cannot harvest and store within themselves the things that are nourishing, that will carry them through periods of austerity? If there is no autumn harvest, the crops that grow in summer will rot where they are without ever being collected and preserved, unable to be used later for food. A person who detests autumn may be having difficulties in harvesting her own energy. This may show as bowel problems like diarrhea, which is an inability to collect the waste for disposal; digestion difficulties like vomiting after eating because the function of gathering nourishment, or harvesting goodness from food, is out of order. Maturity, or harvesting the life experience, is also associated with Metal.

The *Organs* Associated with Metal are the *Lungs* and *Large Intestine*

These are notated as IX for the Lungs, and X for the Large Intestine to avoid confusion between the Western meanings for the anatomical names and the Chinese concepts of a larger sphere of influence than just the organic structure.

According to the *Nei Ching* the Lungs *are the symbol of the interpretation and conduct of the official jurisdiction and regulation.*[4] According to Porkert the Lungs hold the *office of (prime) minister on whom rhythmic order (= specific function) depends.*[5] This function relates to the respiratory functions which affect all the rhythms of the bodymind, not the least of which is the blood flow. Dr. Worsley speaks of the Lungs as the *Official who receives the pure Ch'i from the heavens.* The image which often comes to mind here is that of the infant emerging from the womb into the world and taking that first breath, a moment of moments in the life of humanity. That same breath then carries on as long as the life force flows in us, that is, until death, the last breath. Breathing, though it is something that carries on in spite of ourselves, is one of the main ways we replenish our energy and help the organic functions operate within us. Because it is so simple and basic to life, breathing often gets overlooked, unless a specific symptom like asthma, bronchitis, shortness of breath, or emphysema make us aware of what it means to take air into our lungs. To the Chinese, the function of the Lungs as receiver of energy, taking it from the outside into ourselves, is a function that happens on every level. We breathe emotionally as well as physically. The expressions *breathless with excitement, breathtaking,* refer to that process.

The function of the Large Intestine is spoken of by Dr. Worsley as the *Dust Bin Collector, the Drainer of the Dregs.* The storage and elimination of waste is the main concern of this function. The *Nei Ching* speaks of the Large Intestine as the generator of evolution and change. As every function in the body is *the* most important, so it can be said rightfully that the Large Intestine is the most important function. What would happen if the garbage collector didn't do her job? The garbage would pile up and begin to rot, the people living in the house and their neighbors would begin to complain. The same thing happens within us. If the waste begins to pile up, the rest of the system has to take on an extra load even though it is not equipped to. Feelings of bloatedness, swelling, constipation, emotional stopping up, bad acne and boils, headache and stuffy noise all can point to a malfunctioning of the Large Intestine.

The *Time of Day* for Metal is *Early Morning*

The peak time for the Lungs is from 3:00 A.M.–5:00 A.M., and the peak time for the Large Intestine is from 5:00 A.M.–7:00 A.M. If we were living according to the sun and rising when it does, we would find the natural process of waking up, stretching, deep breathing is truly the beginning of the day. Exercises (like Ti Chi Chuan) are done around 5:00 A.M. in the parks where the air is fresh and the sun is rising. Also, defecation would naturally take place during the hours of Metal. If a person has an imbalance in Metal they may find that this is the worst or in some cases, the best time of day for them.

The *Direction* for Metal is *West*

According to the *Nei Ching precious metals and jade come from the regions of the West* and thus the association. It was also thought that people from the West had a propensity for certain kinds of disease, *ones that strike at the inner body.*[6]

The *Flavor* that Corresponds to Metal is *Pungent, Spicy*

The association of acridity with metal points directly to smelting operations, many of which would give off highly acrid fumes, that is sulphur dioxide.[7] Pungent could refer to cheeses, curry, sauces, peppery sorts of things. A person who craves pungent tastes may very well have a Metal imbalance. An excess of the pungent flavor makes *the muscles become knotty and the fingers and toe nails wither and decay.*[8] *The pungent flavor goes into the respiratory tract; when there is a respiratory tract illness one should not eat too much pungent food.*[9] In further speaking about foods it is said that *when the kidneys suffer from dryness, one should quickly eat pungent food which will moisten them. It will open the pores and bring about a free circulation of the saliva and fluid secretions.*[10]

The *Orifice* and the *Sense Organ* Governed by the Metal Element is the *Nose*

This makes sense when we think of breathing, which we usually do through the nose and the correlation of Lungs with Metal. *The lungs govern the nose.*[11] *White is the color of the West, it pervades the lungs and lays open the nose and retains the essential substances within the lungs.* Many problems which affect the nose have a direct bearing on the Lungs and the Large Intestine, since both are functions within the Metal Element. When we see where the pathway of the Large Intestine is, the relationship of it with the location of the nose makes it clear that nose problems can be associated with the Large Intestine and the whole function of elimination, as well as its association with the Lungs and breathing. Often the sense of smell is affected when the energy in Metal is not properly balanced.

The *Fluid* Secretion Associated with Metal is *Mucous*

Considering the sense organ of Metal, it follows that the secretion of mucous, and the whole of the mucous membranes in the body, as well as in the linings of the air passages, are governed by this Element. Dryness of the throat and nose, coughing, difficulty in breathing, aching in the lungs, raspiness of swallowing and speech problems can be related to the mucous of the body being quantitatively or qualitatively deficient. A person who has a constant nasal drip and a person who has a sinus blockage can, without knowing it, be asking to have the Metal Element, that is the functions of the Lungs and Large Intestine, looked at. Nasal troubles are signals the body uses to let us know whether we are balanced and able to receive energy via breathing.

The *Emotion* Corresponding to Metal is *Grief*

A person who has gone or is going through a period of grief will often have bowel problems and/or breathing difficulties for a while, and sometimes these last a lifetime. The Chinese associated the feeling of deep and prolonged sorrow with the function of the Lungs and the Large Intestine, which comprise the Metal Element. As with each of the emotions, grief is a natural and healthy process, but a person who is overwhelmed by sorrow is likely expressing an imbalance in Metal. On the other hand (and in Chinese thought, there is always another hand), a person who cannot express grief may also be expressing an imbalance in the energy of Metal. *Extreme grief is injurious to the lungs.*[12]

The *Sound* Corresponding to Metal is *Weeping*

This is a natural correspondence to the emotion of grief, yet with some people there is in the voice an unnatural incessant weeping. This is not necessarily accompanied with real tears, but rather is a sound of tears. For these people even happy joyful things are tinged with the sound of weeping. The other hand of this sound is the lack of weeping and the implicit refusal to weep regardless of the situation. This too expresses an imbalance. Listening carefully to the sound of a person's voice can give a clear assessment of the state of the Energy in the Lungs and Large Intestine. The sound of weeping and the emotion of grief coming from a person speak about her ability to receive Energy and the ability to eliminate, both being functions governed by the Metal Element. A person who is always weeping, and to whom tears are ever present, clearly wants help in Metal.

The *Parts of the Body* Governed by the Metal Element are the *Skin* and *Body Hair*

The skin is a third lung and breathes just as surely and necessarily as the lungs themselves. The skin reflects the condition of the Lungs, and the ability to breathe. It is known in Western medicine that many forms of skin problems such as eczema, psoriasis and rashes reflect an imbalance in the body that directly relates to the Lungs. For example, it is not unusual to find asthma accompanied, preceeded or followed by some sort of eczema. This correlation of the skin with the Lungs and respiratory function is an important diagnostic tool to the Chinese, as is that of the other function of Metal. Elimination is also associated with the skin, since the process of getting rid of waste also occurs via the skin. Acne and the other changes during puberty reflect this association; boils and pimples are ways of getting rid of waste from the body via the skin.

The *External Physical* Manifestation of Metal is the *Skin* and the *Body Hair*

Excessive body hair, the loss of body hair, and the lack of body hair (considering the cultural variables) point to Metal. The overall condition of the skin shows the Metal Element's state. *The lungs are connected with the skin. The condition of the body hair shows when the lungs are in splendid and flourishing condition.*[13] Obviously knowing this correlation is a useful diagnostic tool.

The *Power* Granted by Metal is the *Capacity to Cough*

In times of excitement and change.[14] Coughing is associated with mucus being expelled from air passages and also the release of air from the lungs. When there is irritation of the respiratory system, the body expresses this by coughing. On the figurative level, the cough is a rejection of something unwanted, and this capacity to expel something unwanted is associated with Metal and its association with the elimination of waste or unwanted things. This is true emotionally as well as physically.

The *Smell* Associated with Metal is *Rotten*

It is difficult to describe a specific smell accurately in words. Anyone who has worked with sick people knows that, especially with certain diseases like tuberculosis, there is a definite odour of illness. During the traditional examination we assess the odour, which acts as a guide to the imbalance causing illness. If this odour is rotten, we look to the Lungs and the Large Intestine.

The *Climate* Associated with Metal is *Dryness*

Because an excess of any climate is not good for the balance of energy, excessive dryness can affect the energy. If a person does not like a dry climate, or loves a dry climate and cannot stand it otherwise, this may mean the Metal Element wants attention. A person who complains of dryness and whose skin is very dry is also telling us to find out what is happening in Metal. However, a moderately dry climate could be beneficial to someone with a Metal imbalance.

The *Spiritual Resource* Governed by Metal is the *Inferior, Animal Spirit*

It is said that the lungs harbor the animal spirits.[15] I am not sure what is meant by animal spirit, though it could have something to do with the rhythm of breathing and the fact that the plant, insect and animal world share life and breath in common. Everything that is alive breathes, and this breath is controlled by the function of the receiver of Ch'i Energy, the Lungs, which are part of the Metal Element. Breathing puts things in order and keeps them in order. Certainly it is a vital function and controls our most basic (animal?) existence.

Dreams Associated with Metal

The dream motif of Lungs is described by Porkert in translation from the *Nei Ching* and *Ling Shu: white objects* will appear in dreams, or there will be *the cruel killing of people. One will be frightened in dreams, cry, or soar through the air or see strange objects made of metal.*[16] The dreams associated with the Large Intestine are of *fields and rural landscapes.*[17]

The *Other* Correspondences

Associated with Metal is the grain *rice*, the fruit (nut) *chestnut*, the meat *horse*, the vegetable *onions*. All of these foods specifically affect the Element Metal, and these foods combined with all the foods associated with each Element constitute a guide for a healthy balanced diet. If a specific Element is out of balance, the right choice of a food can help restore it.

The number associated with the Element Metal is *nine*. Chinese philosophy refers to the order of generation and the completion of each of the spheres which are referred to as Elements. In this instance the Metal was completed by heaven 9thly and was engendered by earth 4thly.

The musical note of the Element Metal is *shang*. It is said that the musical sounds are manifestations of *talent and ability*. Just what this talent and ability refers to varies from person to person. The musical notes blended together form a harmony of the Elements in sound.

The *Pathways*

The Ch'i Energy flowing in Metal has two pathways. These correspond to the function of the Lungs and the function of the Large Intestine, that is, the receiving of energy via breath, in rhythmic order (the Lungs), and the elimination of waste (the Large Intestine). The Lung pathway begins on the thorax near the clavicle and travels down the inside of the arm and ends at a nail point, IX 11, on the thumb. There are eleven points. This is the external part of the pathway along which the actual points can be treated in order to bring about change and balance within the Metal Element. The functions of reception and elimination on any level can be affected from the points on this meridian. Names like *Cloud Gate, Heavenly Storehouse, Little Merchant* give a clue to the spirit of the Lung meridian and its specific points. A person with a Metal imbalance that shows up as a symptom of asthma or some other sort of congestion of the Lungs may also feel unclear in herself. Using the point *Cloud Gate* might bring balance to the pathway, open the breath and bring clarity to that person. A cloud is an accumulation of congestion; being in the midst of a cloud can feel terribly congested and unstable, like an airplane flying through turbulence. A gate through the cloud, that is, an opening to be able to pass from the haziness, may just be the thing needed in order to lessen the congestion and unclarity. This is what I mean by the *spirit* of a point, and how it speaks to the individual being treated by Acupuncture.

The other pathway in the Metal Element is the Large Intestine. It begins on the nail point of the index finger, travels up the outside of the arm nearly parallel to the Lung Meridian until it ascends over the shoulder along the neck to the face and the nose, where it ends by the side of each nostril. Thus, the connection of the Large Intestine with the nose is evident. Since this pathway controls the function of the elimination of waste, it is relatively easy to see how a needle in one of the 20 points of the Large Intestine Meridian can help in keeping nasal passages clear of waste. Even though this pathway is obviously connected with the nose, it is just as connected with the bowels, although the points affecting the bowels are removed from the actual site. Names like *Joining of the Valleys*, also known as *Harmonious Valley*, and *Support and Rush Out* give us a sense of the power of the Large Intestine pathway. When there is a great disparity within a person, a point like *Joining of the Valleys* can do a tremendous amount to bring balance and harmony to that person. It is, in fact, a powerful point for many imbalances because it joins and connects the Energy within the Metal Element.

The *Pulse*

The pulse of the Lungs is read on the right wrist in the first position at the deep level. The *Nei Ching* states that the feeling of the pulse can give information about the person's illness. For example: *when the pulse of the Lungs beats vigourously and long, the corresponding illness produces blood in the sputum; when the pulse beats are soft and scattered, the corresponding illness produces torrents of sweat which up till the present time cannot be absorbed and issued again.*[18]

The pulse of the Large Intestine is read on the right wrist in the first position at the superficial level. It is the sister Meridian of the Lungs, and together with the reading of the Lung pulse gives us the state of the energy within the Metal Element. By correctly reading the pulses one knows what is happening in all the processes of the human body.

No.	ORGAN/FUNCTION	ELEMENT	YIN/YANG
I	HEART	FIRE	LESSER YIN
II	SMALL INTESTINES	FIRE	GREATER YANG
III	BLADDER	WATER	GREATER YANG
IV	KIDNEYS	WATER	LESSER YIN
V	CIRCULATION/SEX	FIRE	ABSOLUTE YIN
VI	THREE HEATER	FIRE	LESSER YANG
VII	GALL BLADDER	WOOD	LESSER YANG
VIII	LIVER	WOOD	ABSOLUTE YIN
IX	LUNGS	METAL	GREATER YIN
X	COLON	METAL	SUNLIGHT YANG
XI	STOMACH	EARTH	SUNLIGHT YANG
XII	SPLEEN/PANCREAS	EARTH	GREATER YIN

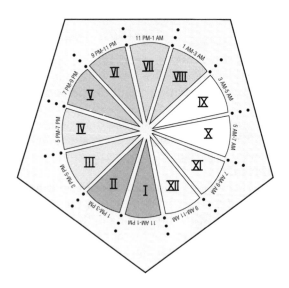

This is adapted with permission from a section of a six-color chart:
The Law of the Five Elements by J.R. Worsley.

Chapter Six

Water

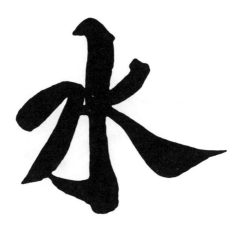

Water

It is wet, fluid; it takes the shape of whatever contains it; it flows; it is essential to life. Water can be cold or warm, murky or clear. It is thirst quenching. It can be supportive and provide a base for travel. It has force and power. It has a rhythm and a cycle. It can be violent and inundating, or it can be serene and submissive. The imagery of water is archetypal—the sea journey, the search for the fountain of youth, the picture of the old watering hole. Watering plants gives them sustenance and nourishment. Water has a refreshing, reinvigorating quality. It is a life principle. Life is unthinkable without water. The human body is about 78% water.

The description of Water in nature is the same description of Water within us. In Chinese terms we *are* the Element Water. We have within us reservoirs, ponds, rivers, seas, oceans of energy, sources of life. Consider the flow of blood, and the river with its tributaries, which we call the blood circulatory system. The lymphatic system is another fluid movement in the body aiding the functions within us; the endocrine fluidity, the urinary fluidity, the fluidity represented by perspiration, saliva, tears, sexual secretions, lactation, all are influenced by the Water Element. If it is not in balance, any aspect of fluidity within our bodymind may go awry. Brittleness of joints, dryness and thirst, frequency or infrequency of urination, excess or deficiency of perspiration, the lack of flow in thought processes and emotions, feelings and fears of inundation, being overwhelmed by things are a few of the symptoms the bodymind can throw up to tell us about an imbalance in the Water Element. An image to use in thinking about the Element Water is a clear sparkling mountain stream circuitously flowing toward a river. If rains come, the stream will swell and become unclear, overflowing its banks. If a drought happens, the stream will decrease and not flow so easily. Should something like a large branch fall across the stream, the water would begin to dam up on one side and merely trickle through on the other side. If the branch is not removed, the stream loses its character and integrity and ceases to be a clear sparkling pathway of flowing water. If this happens within us, we need to know that there is blockage and where to go to remove the block. The key words with the Element Water are fluidity and flow. Wherever that is not happening, we look to Water to see why.

The *Color* Associated with Water is *Blue*

This correspondence is often heard . . . *deep blue sea, blue waters, I feel blue.* A person with a Water imbalance will show blue from the face, especially around the eyes. Often the color preference of this person is blue. If a person's wardrobe is primarily blue, that would lead me to the Water Element. In the classics the color reference for Water is black, and in actuality the hue from the face is a kind of bluish-black. *When their color is black like coal they are without life . . .*[1] Blue is the color most often spoken of as being associated with Water and it is interchangeable with black.

The *Season* That Corresponds to Water is *Winter*

It is often true that a person with a Water imbalance has an aggravation of symptoms in cold weather. A patient who cannot stand the season of winter is probably saying that her Water Element is in trouble. Winter is the time of emphasis; the increased cold seems to crystallize the atmosphere. *All things in creation live shut in and (the crop) is stored away (in winter).*[2] In hibernation, animals go deep into themselves to conserve their essence until the spring. Humans feel inclined to be snuggled cozy and warm in the winter and not to expend much energy. *People should retire early at night and rise late . . .*[3] In fact, the *Nei Ching* speaks specifically about the importance of conserving one's energies in the winter. It is not a time of waste or profligate behavior. It is not a time of extravagance. The snowflake, a symbol of winter, has absolute crystalline economy and beauty, perfect, symmetrical, and whole. Snow covers the earth, protecting the essence of the life which will be reborn in springtime. In terms of human health, this means the preservation of one's own resources and an economizing on the expenditure of energy during the season of winter. If there is an imbalance in the Water Element, this season can be impossible to cope with; symptoms become more pronounced and the cold settles deep into the system. There-fore, nutrition and warmth are important to attend to during winter.

The *Organs* Associated with Water are the *Kidneys* and the *Bladder*

The Roman numeral IV is used for the Kidneys and the Roman numeral III is used for the Bladder. The numbers are used as a universal system in order to avoid translation errors, and to preserve a patient's peace of mind. Reference to a number is not nearly as alarming as reference to an organ name when speaking of malfunc-tioning within the system. If a person hears that III is deficient in energy, she is not nearly as distressed as if she hears that her Bladder is deficient.

According to the *Nei Ching* the Kidneys are *like the officials who do energetic work, and they excel through their ability and cleverness*.[4] Porkert speaks of the Kidneys as an orb or sphere where the basic vital energy has its abode, *The foundation of the native constitution*.[5] Professor Worsley speaks of the Kidneys as the *Storehouse of the Vital Essence* and the *Gateway to the Stomach*. The *Vital Essence* is a way of speaking of the Life Force, especially that aspect of the Life Force that is associated with our very beginnings, the energy we receive from our ancestry. Lethargy characterizes a lack of *Vital Essence*, as do lack of acuity of perception, wishy-washy behavior, and aching in the lower part of the abdomen. These are associated with an imbalance in the Kidneys, which store the *Vital Essence*. The Kidneys regulate the amount of Water in the body. Each cell is comprised of water fluid; fluid bathes the entire cellular system. The flow of the fluid enables waste material to be collected and excreted, in the form of urine. We may very well take this process for granted until something goes wrong with the fluidity of the body that reminds us how fluid is essential to life. The signs may include swelling and bloating, sharp pains, difficulties in urinating, tremendous anxiety, and inability to digest food. It is impossible to take the *Storehouse of the Vital Essence* for granted once we are aware of the functions that depend on proper fluidity. Enormous amounts of blood, about 15 gallons per hour, flow through the Kidneys to be purified and broken down into nutritional components for the body. If the blood does not flow through the Kidneys as it should, symptoms like high blood pressure or hypertension may result, as well as other toxicities that the body would not be able to deal with. *When the Kidneys are deficient . . . the spirit becomes easily provoked . . .*[6]

As the *Gateway to the Stomach*, the Kidneys can be more easily thought of in Chinese terms than in Western terms, for the *Vital Essence* contributes to the process of *rotting and ripening* (see section on Earth, especially description of the Stomach), and to assimilation, nutrition, fruition. A gate is an opening that allows passage from either direction. It is a connector. If the gate is rusty, it becomes unusable; if it is too free, it swings open or closed with the slightest movement. To allow passage it must be flexible, firm, and well-lubricated. The *Vital Essence* lubricates life. A large aspect of life is the digestion and assimilation of the food we take in. The Kidneys allow the stomach to do its job by providing the fluidity and passage of the *Vital Essence*.

The Bladder (III) is spoken of in the ancient texts as an Official of a district which stores *the overflow and the fluid secretions which serve to regulate vaporization.*[7] Porkert refers to the Bladder via translations that clearly ascribe it with the characteristics similar to the Kidneys, and not merely as an excretory organ. Dr. Worsley speaks of the Bladder as the *Official in charge of eliminating fluid waste,* and it is coupled with the function of the Kidney as helping to store the *Vital Essence.* The Bladder is essential to life. If it is not functioning, the rest of the system is stressed beyond endurance and poisoned. It is no little feat to be able to store and eliminate fluid waste from the body and to be flexible enough to contain a little or a lot without great discomfort. Adaptability is a key characteristic of the functioning of the Bladder, and this is significant on every level. A person prone to deep depression, inability to cope with life situations, fears of change, may have an energy imbalance in III, in which the key problem is inability to adapt. Being able to urinate is part of the process of flow within the entire Bodymind-spirit.

The *Time of Day* for Water is *3:00–7:00 P.M.*

This is the peak time for the Energy within the Bladder and the Kidneys. Specifically, the Bladder time is from 3:00–5:00 P.M. and the Kidneys from 5:00–7:00 P.M. A person with an imbalance in Water may find these hours correspond to her lowest time of day. She feels sleepy, droopy, irritable, or anxious. Usually during this time there is an urgency to urinate; the body is saying it wants to empty out, to let go of the waste of the day. A person who feels that this is her best time of day may also be suggesting a slight imbalance in the Water Element because the energy at that time makes her feel just a little bit more alive and excited than usual.

The *Direction* Ascribed to Water is *North*

This makes sense when remembering that the Season ascribed to Water is winter. *The North is the region of storing and laying by.*

The *Climate* Associated with Water is *Cold*

The North is traditionally a cold climate. *The extreme cold causes many diseases. These diseases are most fittingly treated with cauterization by burning the dried tinder of the artemesia (moxa).*[8] There is a good example of the associations made here with the functioning of the Bladder and the Kidneys. When we go outside into the cold during the winter, then back into the house where it is warm, we may have an urgency to urinate. Also, many arthritic problems which arise from a Water imbalance are tremendously affected by cold weather, and usually the pains become more severe and stiffness more intense.

The *Flavor* that Corresponds to the Water Element is *Salty*

It is commonly known that too much salt in the system creates water retention, that people with high blood pressure, which is often associated with the Kidneys even in Western terms, are asked to cut down their intake of salt. A person who eats salt usually has a thirst for fluid. A person who craves salt and uses it excessively is surely asking to check the function of Water within her energy system. The same is true for a person who can *not* stand salt. Joseph Needham in *Science and Civilization in China*, Vol. II, says that *the association of saltiness with water, while natural indeed to a coastal people, suggests primitive experiments and observations on solutions and crystallization.*[9] Other texts refer to the salt taste associated with Water in different ways: *the eating of salt injures the blood.*[10] For this reason the ancient Chinese knew not to eat too much salty food if there were any disease involving the blood. It is said also in the *Nei Ching* the *salty flavor enters into the kidneys.*[11] Salt can feed or aggravate an imbalance in Water.

The *Orifices* Governed by the Water Element are the *Genitals*, the *Urethra*, and the *Anus*

A great deal of sexual functioning depends on the balance within the Element Water. The health of reproduction, the workings of the testicles and the ovaries, the flow of energy needed in the sexual act, as well as the lubrication not only of the sperm but also of the egg, depend on a balanced Water Element. The medium of life for the embryo is Water. Often sexual problems are directly attributable to an imbalance in this Element—problems including impotence, frigidity, sterility. There are specific points on the Bladder and the Kidneys'Meridian that are directly linked with sexual function and reproduction.

The *Sense Organ* Governed by the Water Element is the *Ears*

We also spoke about the ears in connection with the Fire Element, but that was more to do with the orifice of the ears governed by Fire, rather than the sense organ. The association of the ears with Water has more to do with the sense of hearing itself. One of the earliest sense faculties developed is hearing, and as I have mentioned, early embryonic development and the aquatic milieu of the developing baby are closely linked with the development of the Kidneys. The ear is shaped like an inverted embryo, and Acupuncture points on the ear correspond to the embryonic organ development. Another correlation of Water with hearing is the ability to hear sounds underwater. Liquid is part of the hearing process. The fluid in the canals is controlled by the Water Element. Symptoms like vertigo, dizziness, loss of equilibrium and balance, and noises like the sound of a waterfall can be the result of an imbalance of energy within the Water Element.

The *Fluid Secretion* Associated with Water is *Saliva,* or *Spittle*

The Chinese thought of saliva as two distinct secretions produced and related to two different Elements, Earth and Water. The saliva associated with Water has to do with the teeth, because the teeth are governed by the Water Element. The lubrication in our mouth is absolutely essential to the process of eating, digesting and speaking. Though we are usually not aware of it, the teeth are always wet, bathed in saliva. Dryness of the mouth, oversecretion of saliva, drooling, these could be symptoms related to the secretion associated with Water. A baby who is teething drools and dribbles saliva from the mouth, and her urine becomes stronger in concentration. This illustrates another connection between Water associations.

The *Emotion* Associated with Water is *Fear*

Extreme fear is injurious to the kidneys, but fear can be overcome by contemplation.[12] Phobias of all sorts fall within this category of fear: that is, fear of heights, of water, of people, of new things, of sexuality, of closed spaces, of the dark, of death. It is not only these extreme fears that tell us there is an imbalance in Water: it can also be a general amorphous feeling of dread or foreboding, a pervading sense of anxiety about life. This association of fear with the Water Element sheds some light on the origins of insanity and the desires to commit suicide. Simplistically, fear can be thought of as a holding on, rather than a flow and letting go of things that we feel anxious about. If the energy is flowing well, we can experience life like the flow of a river; if it is not flowing well, we experience life like a nightmare, feeling overwhelmed, inundated, sinking into dispair.

The *Sound* that Corresponds to Water is *Groaning*

Another description of this sound is moaning or humming. This is pervasive in the person who has imbalances within Water. Her voice continually moans and groans, even though her life is no more problem-ridden than average. The sound happens in spite of herself.

The *Parts of the Body* Governed by the Water Element are the *Bones* and the *Bone Marrow*

Our human skeleton, that is, the framework which provides us with form, movement and protection, is governed by the Water Element. This means bones everywhere, including the teeth, the skull, the spinal column, the limb and torso bones, are kept strong and rigid by being fed via the energy of the Bladder and Kidney functions. The functions performed by the Kidneys and the Bladder extend beyond the actual anatomical structure of the organs. For example, fluidity and force are the properties of Water directly linked with the Kidneys and Bladder and therefore connected with the bones in the body. The marrow is included as part of the bone because it is within the bone that cells are formed which nourish and give strength and replacement, continually renewing the person. Also, because the brain is considered the *sea of marrow* it is thus governed by the Water Element. Problems with bones anywhere in the body are connected with a malfunctioning of this Element. *The kidneys harbor the force of life of the bones and marrow.*[13]

The *External Physical* Manifestation of the Water Element is the *Head Hair*

To assess the condition of the energy within the Water Element one would look at the hair on the head, feel its texture and growth, and determine whether it is brittle, dry, broken, or split. Many cases of balding, partial or total in men and women, have to do with an imbalance of Water. In a person whose hair is falling out, there are often other symptoms which also belie a Water imbalance. One man, who was being treated because of the symptoms of asthma and high blood pressure, began to have his hair grow back during the course of treatment.

The *Power* Granted by Water is the *Capacity to Create Trembling*

In times of excitement and change. Trembling is often a release, a letting go of tightness and pent-up tensions, even when it is accompanying chronic illness. Anyone who has ever experienced strong fear has also experienced the accompanying trembling or shaking, as is a natural response to tension. If, however, there is excess trembling, one would look immediately to the Water Element to see whether the energy is balanced.

The *Smell* Associated with Water is *Putrid*

One would expect that this smell would connect with the smell of urine since urine is so directly linked to Water, yet the odour described as putrid is more acrid and putrefied than urine. It is quite distinct, though not easily described. In most instances the odour is subtle, but in cases of bad Kidney and Bladder problems the smell is quite strong. Even a hint of this odour suggests an imbalance in the Water Element.

The *Spiritual Resource* Governed by the Water Element is *Will Power* and *Ambition*

It is said that the Kidneys harbor these.[14] It is also said that the Kidneys *call to life that which is dormant and sealed up; they are the natural organ for storing away . . .*[15] Everyone knows what it means to have will power or the lack of it and almost everyone knows what it means to want to achieve something. The force propelling a person toward actually doing something comes from the clarity within the Water Element. If this clarity is not there, a person can suffer from lack of personal force in life and get buffeted around by other people's strength and will. A person lacking will power is expressing a symptom of a Water imbalance as clearly as a person who has cystitis or sexual problems.

The *Dreams* Associated with Water

The dream motifs of Water as related by Porkert[16] translated from the Chinese texts are: dreams of *ships, boats, drowning people, lying in the water and being frightened, the sensation of the back and waist split apart and can no longer be stretched, approaching a ravine, plunging into the water, or being in the water.* Dreams specifically associated with the Bladder are of taking walks and excursions.[17]

The *Other* Correspondences

The foods associated with Water are: the fruit, *dates;* the grain, *beans and peas;* the animal, *pig;* and the vegetable, *leeks.* According to Porkert the scaley animals, that is, the fishes, are also associated with Water. These foods, like the foods associated with all the other Elements, are only meant to be a guideline to a balanced diet.

The number associated with the Element Water is *six*. According to the philosophy of the Chinese, Water was engendered first by heaven and completed sixth by Earth, thus the association of the number six with the Element Water. Often a person has a favorite number and equally often this preference coincides with the particular imbalance of that person. This not to say that if a person's favorite number is six she has a Kidney or Bladder problem!

The musical note associated with the Water Element is *yu*, or the sound of the twenty-five stringed lute. Music is a manifestation of the harmony of life and the energy flowing throughout the universe. The combination of these sounds expresses this harmony. Like the sounds of an orchestra the notes sweep together with spirit and skill to form a unified whole. The Five Elements work together like an orchestra.

The *Pathways*

The Ch'i Energy of Water flows in two pathways. These pathways correspond to the Bladder and the Kidneys and control the functioning of them. The Bladder is the largest meridian of the whole body. It has 67 Acupuncture points. The pathway begins at the inside corner of the eye, travels up over the head, down the neck, down along the back parallel to the spinal column, down to the bottom of the spine, back up along the spine again in a line parallel to the spinal column, then down along the back of the leg, to the back of the knee, down the calf, then the outside of the leg, ending at the nail point of the little toe, on the outside of the nail. Looking at this meridian and thinking of the correspondences of the Water Element, for example, the association of bones with Water, we see that the pathway of the Bladder covers the whole body, especially the back area along the vertebral column. It is a very important pathway. There are certain points on it which affect the functioning of all the other organs in the body in a direct and powerful way. Many illnesses, even of chronic duration, have been cured using the points of the Bladder Meridian. The point names indicate the spirit of the Bladder Meridian, that is, *Spirit Hall, Thought Dwelling, Penetrating the Valley, Eyes Bright.*

The pulse of the Bladder is read on the left hand in the third position at the superficial level. It is the sister pulse of the Kidneys and tells what the energy is like in Water throughout the system. Considering the length of the pathway, the quality and quantity of energy is given great attention.

The other pathway of the Water Element is that of the Kidneys. This begins on the bottom of the foot, comes up over the ankle on the inside of the foot, travels up the leg to the knee on the inside, then up to the abdomen along the groin, up along the torso in a line parallel to the midline of the body, and ends on the clavicle. It has 27 points, and like all the other pathways described, it is bilateral and symmetrical. Looking at the actual path of the meridian on the body, we can see its connection with the sexual self. Points like *Bubbling Spring, Blazing Valley, Greater Mountain Stream, Great Cup, Ch'i Cave, Vitals Correspondence, Dark Gate* describe the vital essence housed by the Kidneys. Other names are more connected with the spirit, like *Spirit Seal, Spirit Wilderness, Spirit Storehouse,* and give the sense of dealing directly with a person's intimate inner self. Inasmuch as these names suggest dealings on an emotional and spiritual level, it would be a shame to overlook their significance.

The *Pulse*

The pulse of the Kidneys is read in the third position on the left hand at the deep level of energy.

> *When the pulse of the kidneys stops beating and becomes interrupted as though fingers were snapped upon stone and swerved ... death strikes.*[18]

> *At the point of death the pulse of the kidneys flows and makes itself manifest like the tearing of twisted cord or like the snapping of fingers upon stone ...*[19]

> *The pulse of the kidneys should sound like a stone (that is, according to Wang Ping: It should sound deep and strong like a stone thrown).*[20]

The Ch'i Energy, that is, the Life Force, should be flowing pure and clear in every pulse, in a balanced harmonious way. By feeling the pulses we can know if this is happening and if it is possible to help it flow in a more clear and balanced way.

Section Two

Chapter Seven

Traditional Examination

The Location of the Pulses

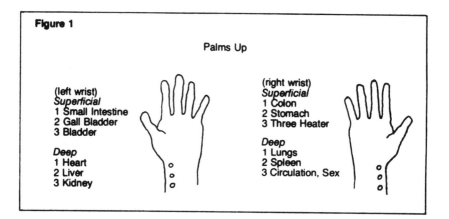

Figure 1

Palms Up

(left wrist)
Superficial
1 Small Intestine
2 Gall Bladder
3 Bladder

Deep
1 Heart
2 Liver
3 Kidney

(right wrist)
Superficial
1 Colon
2 Stomach
3 Three Heater

Deep
1 Lungs
2 Spleen
3 Circulation, Sex

Traditional Examination

To See, To Hear, To Ask, To Feel

The examination for Traditional Acupuncture has four major tenets—to see; to hear; to ask; to feel. This is done using the perceptions and skills of a 5,000-year-old tradition. The examination is the basis for diagnosis. What I want to do is present the process so that those who know little about Traditional Acupuncture will have an understanding of it. I will go through the examination step by step, the way a Traditional Acupuncturist would to gather enough information to diagnose the causative factor of a person's illness. Some of the information asked is familiar to those who have visited a Western physician. Although much of the examination may make no sense from a Western viewpoint, the Traditional Oriental approach to the human being reveals valuable insights. There is nothing a patient says or does that is not important to her own personal health. Hopefully this becomes clear to the patient during the course of the examination.

As a person comes through the door to be examined, the first thing that is noticed is her demeanor, gait, the colors predominant in her appearance, the hues coming from her face (in natural light), and the mannerisms of her person. It is important to remember that no judgements are made about the patient. The most important thing in the whole process of examination is accurate recording and the reflection of what the entirety of the patient is saying. This is done with as much clarity on the part of the practitioner as possible. It is not *bad* if the patient is wearing all blue, or talking loudly, or walking stiffly, or any other possible variations.

Introductions are made between the patient and Acupuncture practitioner. In England first names are almost always used unless a patient prefers to call the practitioner by a surname or be called by a surname. Each person is asked what she would like to be called. This procedure is basic and essential to establish a relationship. We must learn to work together in an integral and intimate way, integral because the human being cannot be dichotomized and still be whole, intimate because the depth to which the patient and practitioner must go in order to establish health and harmony is often the deepest relationship a person has.

In the treatment room, the practitioner physically contacts the patient for the first time, usually via a handshake. A hand extended outward speaks to the world. It expresses the fears, desires, and inner feelings of the person who has come for help. Often it is the handshake that tells what the patient is *asking* for. Therefore, not only the grip, but the texture, temperature, moisture and duration are all important.

The patient and practitioner sit together talking about things like correct spelling of name, address, how to be contacted, phone number, and who referred the patient to the clinic. This is the time for finding out what sort of work a person does, whether she is active, sedentary, whether there is any stress of a physical or emotional nature in her work. Oftentimes occupational hazards cause the patient to react in a compensatory way without realizing it; that is, a bus conductor carrying the money change gear around his neck is weighted down in front, which puts stress on other parts of his body; a person who has an office job with responsibility for 25 other people carries stress somewhere in order to cope with the job. If I sound simplistic in some examples, I assure you that it is often the simplest and most obvious that directs the Acupuncture practitioner to clearly see the totality of the person asking for help.

What is your age, date, time and place of birth? This information gives an idea of life experience as well as the facts about the birth. A patient often has second-hand information about what was happening around the time she was born and what sort of birth it was. The place, for example—near the water, in the mountains, or in the city, can determine environmental influences upon a person. The exact time gives access to phases of the planets which, although not necessary, may be used as adjunct information. It is also true that a person born at a particular season may express an imbalance in the Element correlated with that season. For example, a person who is born in Autumn may have a tendency toward a Metal imbalance in which the Lungs or Large Intestine may be affected. These correlations are drawn out clearly in the chapters on the Five Elements. The above does *not* mean that because a person was born in Autumn she therefore has asthma and is constipated. It only *may* mean that she *might* have difficulty associated with those two organs. I want to be very careful to give qualified information at each step of this process, because nothing is one-sided in Acupuncture. I can not make a general statement that is forever true; I can only give you a framework through which to see some of the myriad possibilities.

With whom do you live? Within this question lies a great deal of day-to-day life information about the patient; husband, wife, man, woman, parents, children, friend, stresses, burdens, joys, expectations, and tensions are discussed. Often the roles in a home situation harbor clues to illness. However, so early in an examination one can not always have built enough trust to be able to unlock those areas. There are other places in the course of the examination to gather more information.

Why are you coming to the clinic? This question asks about the main thing that is wrong. It elicits information on the concrete, most troubling symptom, whatever it might be. The answer often is given in the form of a label, e.g. migraine, insomnia, asthma, arthritis, frigidity, diarrhea, polyneuralgia, dyspnoea, high blood pressure, diabetes, and so on. However, as a label, none of these is important to the Traditional Acupuncture practitioner. I want to know what is the experience of the trouble, to hear a description of when, how, where it happens to *you.* Describe it in the context of your life: when did it begin, what was happening at the time, does it have a color, a temperature, where exactly does it being, how does it end, does it ever end, how do you cope with it, and do you have any hunches about what it is connected with? This is not a question with a specific answer. It is rather a chance for the patient to reflect and roam around her own head for the experience of the problem. The label tells nothing specific about the individual suffering. I need to know the history, the context, the description. Does anything help it? Do you have anything the trouble is related to? Everything the patient says here, word for word, is recorded the way it is said. For example, one patient said, *I worked in a museum where it was damp and cold. I sat in a polished chair for nearly seven years. I had a fall off that chair because I was wearing a nylon overall. It must have been slippery. My tail started to ache, then my left leg and hip got very painful, a shocking, sharp pain. I suffered it and didn't tell anyone. I'm like that, I'm afraid. I couldn't sleep. It was driving me mad. I think I have a weakness in my heart.* She said this matter-of-factly with a smile on her face, even though she was in pain as she spoke.

At this point I am collecting everything I see and hear, jotting things I want to query in a separate place so that I can return there if I need more information. The above is an excerpt from a woman patient who came in saying *I have arthritis.* What I have given you is a brief, incomplete portion of her own description of the arthritis.

Any other problems or complaints? Are there things you might not ordinarily go to a doctor for? This question opens the possibility of finding out what else is troubling to a person even though it might have been something she would not have ordinarily mentioned. Things like: I have difficulty in making decisions, my ring finger often has pins and needles, I am angry a lot, my eyes feel watery, I am often cold in the extremities, I feel like moaning all the time are some examples of other things wrong. In Traditional Acupuncture *every* symptom, everything a person has to say about herself is important and taken into consideration. Each of us is a unique combination of humanity. It is often a relief to a person to discover that she is being taken seriously regardless of how mundane or unusual her problem.

What is your medical history? Have you had any surgery, any accidents, diseases, or hospitalizations? The answer to this question gives an historical chronological perspective on a person's health. It also tells what surgery has been done and which meridians have been cut across and where. Were there any side or after effects? If there have been accidents or injuries, which parts of the body were most affected? If there were diseases, what order did they come in, and how severe were they? This answer often gives a relative guide to the path the Law of Cure will take. The body *remembers* and carries within itself the remnants of past illness, especially if that illness was palliated and not allowed to take its full course. In the process of healing, the patient often will get a return, a sort of glimpse at the old illness as it passes from the bodymind. For example, asthma from childhood may return for an hour or two and then be gone for good. Depression in younger years, feelings of dread, even an old fear of the dark may come back momentarily as it passes. This is not always so, but knowing the history of illness can give a clue to the healing process for an individual.

What is your family medical history?—that of your parents, brothers, sisters, grandparents, sons, daughters, spouse? This section of the examination provides information about hereditary and constitutional factors. Often a patient has a worry that what happened to her parents may happen to her; she may worry about things like diabetes, a nervous breakdown, cancer, or arthritis. This is reason enough to find out the family medical history. Any worry a person has is important. Often life patterns, attitudes, frames of reference for a world view are repeated from generation to generation. This is true too for tendencies toward certain energy imbalances. But because there may be tendencies toward certain patterns does not mean that a person cannot avoid that route. It does mean, though, that it is important to know those tendencies.

What is your emotional history? How were you as a child? Did you have any difficulties that can be remembered; any strong features? How did you get along with others, how did you feel growing up? Was there any trauma in childhood, like moving or a family death, that was terribly upsetting? These are important to know because the past remains within us. Many of our adult fears are compounded upon childhood fears that were never dealt with. And not just fear, but anger, joy, compassion, grief, in fact, all the emotions as we experienced them stay with us and affect us now. Every imbalance we have now is associated with some emotion. Every illness, every symptom is connected with an emotion. (This is discussed in detail in the chapters on the Five Elements.)

How would you describe yourself emotionally? This question concentrates on the present tense, the emotions a person may have most difficulty in dealing with. Usually a person is aware of an emotion that is difficult to express, or one that is foremost. Often there is a great gap between feeling and acting. It encourages a description of how we really feel inside, even if for years we have been fooling others. This self-description is a focus for a patient to begin to see how emotions are connected with all of life. This section may hit upon difficulties in relationships very specific to the patient's emotional needs in the present. This question gives strong clues to the state of the energy in all the Elements.

What is your favorite color? This is a question that recognizes a connection between color and illness as seen by the Chinese, rarely seen by the Western physician. Blue goes with the Element Water, which corresponds to the pathways of Energy of the Bladder and the Kidney. This does not mean that just because blue is your favorite color therefore your bladder is diseased. It may mean that your Water Element needs to be nourished, to be brought into harmony with the other Elements. If you hate the color blue, this may be as significant a sign of imbalance as if you love the color blue. Either way *may* be saying *check out my Bladder and Kidney meridians.* More often than not, a patient is surprised to hear herself saying *I hate red, or blue or green, etc.* with a vehemence she did not know she had. Often too the patient realizes that the clothes she buys and the environment surrounding her is strongly predominated by one color, sometimes temporarily, sometimes permanently. I hesitate to say this for fear of self-diagnosis on the part of the reader and little bits of paranoia lest you love some color and loathe another. There is no judgment. Every single thing about us points to and speaks to the entirety. We can see the connections and bring about balance where it has gone askew. The information gathered via traditional diagnosis gives us what we need to find health again.

What season do you like or not like? Each season corresponds to an Element. Autumn is associated with the Element Metal. The two organ systems related to Metal are the Lungs and Large Intestine. If you hate Autumn, you may be asking someone to find out if the energy in your Metal Element is balanced and in harmony with the rest. The same could be true if you love Autumn to the exclusion of the other seasons. Though there are not always exact correlations to be made, more often than not, the Chinese have made accurate predictions regarding the seasons and illness.

What climate do you like best, or not like at all? It is important to note that everything in Acupuncture may mean one thing and its opposite. What is intensely liked or disliked points to the same thing. Heat is associated with the Element Fire and the season of Summer. This corresponds to the meridians of the Heart and the Small Intestines, as well as the pathways of the Three Heater and Circulation Sex, two functions unknown to Western medicine. If you hate a warm climate, cannot stand the heat, or if you love it and cannot stand the cold, you may be asking us to check the balance of the energy in your Fire Element, that is, your Heart, Small Intestines, Three Heater and Circulation Sex.

What time of day do you feel better or worse? To the Traditional Acupuncturist this question relates to the Chinese bodyclock, which relates to the time of peak energy in each of the Elements during a 24-hour period. The Element Wood, for example, is at its height of energy from 11:00 P.M. to 3:00 A.M. This means that during this time the energy in the Gall Bladder Meridian and the Liver Meridian is just that much fuller than in the other pathways. If a patient says she feels much better at this time of night, better than at any other time, this may be a signal to check if Wood is in trouble. On the other hand, as I have already said, the alternate may be just as significant. If a person feels worse than at any other time, again we would query the Element. According to the Chinese, every hour of the day carries one of our organic functions a little more strongly than the others. Because this follows a natural bodily rhythm, the body will let us know when something is not right.

What is your favorite taste? Is there something that you really do not like the taste of? Taste often works as a gauge to show that the body harmony is beginning to deteriorate. Since food is the sustenance of life, it makes sense that everything about it is relevant to the energy we have. Thus, the importance of taste. There are five categories of taste, each corresponding to one of the Elements. Sweet is the flavor associated with the Element Earth. The Element Earth is associated with the meridian of the Stomach and the meridian of the Spleen-Pancreas. We know that there are people who have a *sweet tooth*, people who have to have a chocolate bar every day and who cannot pass up a pastry shop. And there are the rarer ones who never eat sweets, who, in fact, intensely dislike sweets. Does this mean that their Stomachs are in trouble or that their Spleens are malfunctioning? Not necessarily, but to the trained person who correlates all the information from the examination, the food preferences suggest the meridians that may need more balance. This is not as simple as it first sounds. According to the laws within the Law of the Five Elements, the Earth Element may be the one most obvious in signaling distress, but it may not be the one causing the problem. Each Element depends on the Element preceding it, forming an interdependent harmonized network among all Five, like friends living happily in the same house with only minor ups and downs.

The following part of the examination is usually known as the *review of systems*. It is familiar to Western medicine though some of the correlations are different. I will explain to you as clearly as I can how each step is relevant to the Traditional Acupuncture practitioner in determining someone's state of health.

How is your head? Does it ever ache? Do you ever feel dizzy? This question focuses the patient's attention on a very important part of herself. Most of us spend a lot of time in our heads, often to the exclusion of the rest of our bodies and, I might add, to the detriment of our heads. When anything begins to go wrong, the head is often the place that bears the brunt or acts as a radar for the rest of our innerself. Tension traditionally is borne there, as television commercials attest. Most of us have something to say about our heads, or, at least, can begin to take cognizance of how our heads are connected to the rest of ourselves. The description that a person gives can be a guide to the cause of the difficulty.

Do you wear spectacles, or any sort of corrective lenses? Are you long or short sighted? Do your eyes burn, feel grainy, or get unusually red? Have you noticed any change in them lately? Most of this kind of information comes up in the first part of the examination when asking about other complaints, other than the main one. Often though, it is forgotten and this *review of systems* can bring it out. Eyes are governed by the Element Wood, and therefore whatever is happening with the eyes may be saying something specific to that Element, and to the meridians of the Gall Bladder and Liver, which belong to that Element. Frequently a patient's vision improves during the course of Acupuncture treatment as the energy becomes balanced. This is important because even though the main symptom may be still present, there are ways for the patient to experience improvement. Imagine the pleasure of hearing from your optometrist that your eyesight has improved. In instances where a chronic condition, such as what is labeled arthritis, will take a long time to be put right, the patient needs to know that something in her world is improving concretely.

How are your ears? Do you hear well? Ears are an often overlooked part of our daily life. What we hear and how we hear it is a sense that puts us in or out of contact with other human beings. The caricature of the elderly deaf person trying to hear what someone else is saying and then repeating something entirely different is not a funny one. Music, laughter, all the sounds of the universe are experienced through our ears, as well as the noises and the voices of those we'd rather not listen to—the sounds of the human condition. There is much lore and some fact about the shape of the ear being connected with our fetal development, the ear itself being an upside down fetus configuration. Acupuncture points on the ear are said to correspond to the development and the location of the organs within this figure. This is the reason why staple puncture for weight loss centers on the ear. This is a dangerous form of symptomatic acupuncture which does not take the wholeness of the patient into consideration. A person who has had lots of ear problems, like ringing, buzzing, aching, burning, may be suggesting that the Water Element or the Fire Element needs some attention.

How is your nose? How is your sense of smell, how are your breathing passages? Do you get nosebleeds? Noses, like ears, are caricatured and underestimated. There is often a great deal of emotion and concern surrounding the image of our noses. *Nose jobs* are not uncommon. Categories are set up such as aquiline, schnozzer, snub, and pug to label the image. Yet, the function of the nose, which is to smell, is often overlooked. The state of energy in the Earth functions, i.e., the stomach and spleen, is related directly to the nose. Another function of the nose is to get rid of debris. Because of this it is also closely connected with the Large Intestine, the eliminator, a function within the Element Metal. In fact, the last point on the Large Intestine meridian is just to the side of the nose and is called *Welcome Fragrance.*

How is your mouth? Is there a history of dental trouble, soft teeth, extractions? Sore throats, strept throat, tonsillitis, adenoids, any problems to do with the mouth and passage? Are there tastes that are not clear to you? Can you distinguish salt, sour, bitter? Are there any speech difficulties? Our mouths control one of our main sources of energy, production, i.e., food and drink. Mastication, which takes place here, is the beginning of the process of nourishment.

How is your skin? Is it dry; does it bruise easily; do you have any rashes? Skin is our outer covering. We take in and give out through it. The Chinese consider it the Third Lung. It is a protective covering that extends to the world. *Thick-skinned, thin-skinned, skinny, the skin of his teeth* refer to this extension of ourselves. Skin is governed by the Metal Element, the Lungs and the Large Intestine. This makes almost immediate sense when you think that the skin breathes through its pores, and that it gives off waste in the form of perspiration. It is via the skin and the pathways of energy that run along it that we do Acupuncture because the Acupuncture points are located there.

How are your hair and scalp? Head hair is governed by the Water Element, and so the condition of hair and scalp is giving information about the Bladder and Kidneys. The hair of a person who is sick often goes through changes, like hair loss, dryness of scalp, excess of oiliness and color change.

How are your nails? Nails are governed by the Element Wood. If they are ridged, brittle, soft, splitting, or discolored, this could be the bodymind's reflection on the condition of the Liver and Gall Bladder, the two organs within the Element Wood. The nails on the feet as well as on the hands tell the condition of the Wood Element. However, it is not always true that someone who has an imbalance in the Wood will have fingernails that show this. Although the patient may point us in the direction of the cause of illness, one sign that fits does not necessarily mean we have the answer. A very involved correlation of *all* the information is the only way an accurate diagnosis is made.

How are your bones? Oftentimes a patient knows about her bones, that is, whether or not something is wrong. *I feel it in my bones* is an old weather gauge. Bones are governed by the Water Element (this involves the Bladder and the Kidneys) whose season is winter, traditionally a time when bone problems become acute, for example, in many people with arthritis. People prone to bone injuries (fractures, and breaks) are often those with a Water imbalance.

How are your muscles? Patients often have something to say about their muscles, whether they are flaccid, weak, strong, spastic, cramping, or out of shape and tone. According to the Chinese, Earth governs the muscles in the human body.

How is your urination? This question asks for all the aspects of getting rid of waste fluid. It covers frequency, control, color, odor, history of urogenital infections, burning, discharge, retention, and time of day when any of these is more prominent. Though the Bladder is the organ most in charge of the urinary function, and thus, by association the Water Element, including the Kidneys, the flow of waste from the body may have much to do with several other functions. For example, it may be the Spleen which transports, the Large Intestine which throws out debris, or the Small Intestine which sorts. Attaching these functions to these organs is an Eastern concept and not easily translated into Western concepts of organ function.

Do you perspire? Perspiration follows the question on urination since both are the body's natural way of dispensing waste fluids. Some people never perspire, some perspire all the time; one may have nightsweats that are not salty, another has night sweats that are salty; another may perspire only at certain times of day; someone else may perspire only at certain spots. There are many variations and all are significant.

How are your bowels? Is there a tendency toward diarrhea or constipation? (This affects the emotions.) Is there regularity, if so, when? What upsets the pattern? Is there a great deal of flatulence? What color are the stools? Do they float? Do you have hemorrhoids, pruritis ani, any lesion or rectal fissure? The whole excretory function is governed by the Large Intestine, which is a function within the Metal Element. Although the condition of the bowels asks us to have a look at Metal, to say that the bowels are only and always connected with the Large Intestine is not true. In fact, Water as the Element of flow and lubrication sometimes has as much to say about the bowels as does Metal.

How do you sleep? How many hours—from when til when? Do you wake up tired? Sleep is itself a healer of the bodymind. For too many people natural sleep, that is sleep without medication, is rare. The high stress of daily living and internal turbulence often rob people of this essential healer. Exhaustion that finds no recompense in sleep is compounded and deepened, forcing the bodymind to cope without the necessary resources. Even a little sleep problem wreaks havoc in a person's life. Sleep, like food and breathing, is something that affects and is affected by the balance of all the Elements. How a patient describes her sleep is a direct key to the Element most in trouble.

Do you dream? Is there any recurrent theme? This information follows the question about sleep to find out the Element most needing attention. Specific subjects of dreams, like *uncultivated fields*, are spoken of in the indications for certain Acupuncture points. The whole subject of dreaming gives data about ourselves that we are usually not aware of, information about our fears and desires, our traumas and catastrophic expectations, our self-images and creative blocks. This question does not involve dream analysis, but rather images which give leads on specific imbalances.

Do you smoke? How many cigarettes per day? How many pipefulls of tobacco, how many cigars? The fact that the question is even asked is significant. It is obvious to people who smoke and to others who warn people not to smoke that nicotine alters a person's system. The Lungs and the blood stream are affected, but the habit is even more insidious and subtle, partly just because it is a habit that a human being has come to depend on and goes through trauma trying to break. It is important to know if a person smokes and to what extent, how they feel about it, and whether they are trying to stop.

Do you drink? What do you drink and how much? This question asks the amount of fluid intake daily, and what it is, tea, coffee, water, milk, alcohol, juice, soda, or other beverages. The Element Water has most to do with the control of fluid in the body. The amount of liquid we take in affects Water, e.g., bloating, dehydration, dry-brittleness. It is not unusual to find a direct correlation between a person who feels parched and the lack of liquid intake, though this is not always true. Someone can feel very dry and be drinking 20 cups of something per day. If the liquid is tea or coffee, it is important to know how much sugar is taken. One or two teaspoons per cup at 12 cups per day is a sizeable amount of sugar. Though more nutritional than refined sugar, honey can also be excessive in this amount, especially for people who are trying to control their weight.

What is your diet? What do you eat and how much? Do you enjoy it? Are you following a regime? How do you decide what to eat? What are you most attracted to? The reverse of the old saying *eat to live, don't live to eat* bombards our senses constantly. The quick food stands and supermarkets offer foods of questionable nutritional value and unquestionable appeal. What we take in as the sustenance of our lives determines how we feel, act, look, and think. If what we take in is balanced, it contributes to our balance. A simple inspection of daily food often shows the patient that she is just not nourishing herself properly, and so she feels sluggish, fat, or low in energy and vitality. Diet is one of the main ways we help ourselves stay alive and healthy. If certain things are missing, like vitamins, minerals and proteins, the Acupuncturist must guide a person not toward a regimented diet, but to a balanced one.

Do you take any medications? This question includes vitamins, dietary supplements, laxatives, the birth control pill, aspirin and prescriptions of any sort. Certain drugs are known to have side effects and carry special precautions or contraindications. A drug for an arthritic problem may very well affect the Water Element severely. Wood is also often put out of balance. Tranquilizers fool the bodymind, and though they may be necessary in certain instances, are often throwing a natural balance even further off. The fewer drugs a person takes, the better off the person is. In bodymind we want to be healthy and balanced, and as we seek this via Acupuncture, the drug may be a deterrent to real health. In treatment, we would try, if at all possible, to gradually lower the dosage until a person can function without medication. Sometimes this just is not possible because the dependence on drugs is such that the body can no longer perform its own functions without help. One difficult question in the midst of medication is the use of the birth control pill. There are very few women on the pill whose pulses do not show an imbalance directly related to the birth control pill. However, the tension and the heartache of not having the protection of the pill often create more imbalance in the energy.

What is your menstrual cycle like? What age did it begin? Are you regular? How long does it last; is there any discomfort, depression, or changes? Is it a heavy flow? When was your last period? Have you ever been pregnant? What was the pregnancy like, and the birth? Do you desire to be pregnant? The rhythmic cycle of life, fulfillment of sexuality and procreation are governed by the Water, Fire and Earth Elements. This is true of men and women. In fact, the Ch'i Energy that governs the menstrual cycle also governs a cycle in men. There are rhythm and flow of Life Force in *all* human beings.

How is your general energy level? Do you feel like you have enough energy, or so much that you cannot relax? How is your sexual energy? Acupuncture treatment deals directly with the movement and balance of Ch'i Energy. This question asks a person to describe her own Energy. One of the most bound-up of personal places is the area of sexuality. Every relationship at some point entertains sex. It is inextricably woven into our lives, though often not integrated, wholesomely experienced and enjoyed. Tension, cutting off of desire, and images of performance characterize a great deal of it. The Life Force within us seeks to flow freely and if it is not flowing gives us a sign that there is a blockage. If a person has a problem sexually, that is an important sign of an energy imbalance, yet sexual needs too often go unmentioned in the discussion of illness or health. It is important to internal harmony that we listen to what the body-mindspirit is telling us.

To Feel

This part of the discussion of an examination revolves around the fourth tenet of traditional diagnosis, that is, to feel. Because the understanding of this depends so heavily on familiarity of the twelve pulses, I will begin this section with a description of what the pulses are.

> *Hence it is said: Those who wish to know the inner body feel the pulse and have thus the fundamentals for diagnosis.*[1]

There are twelve main paths of energy in the body. These are called Meridians, and they correspond to the twelve main functions of the body. Ten of these functions are named after the ten major organs of the body; they are the Heart, the Small Intestines, the Bladder, the Kidneys, the Gall Bladder, the Liver, the Lungs, the Large Intestine, the Stomach and the Spleen (Pancreas).

The two functions are Circulation Sex and Three Heater. Their place in the order above is between the Kidneys and the Gall Bladder. This order is notated in Roman numerals, beginning with I for the Heart and ending with XII for the Spleen (Pancreas). I say this because we record the pulses in Roman numerals on the examination form. Because this system is international, it avoids errors in word translation: errors that could be dangerous to patients.

Each of these twelve functions has a pathway which could be thought of as a river of energy continuously flowing through the body. Illness is the bodymind's way to say that one or more of these pathways does not have the proper amount or the correct quality of energy flowing through it. How do we find out which one? The pulse of each pathway can be felt along any major artery of the body. We usually use the wrist pulses over the radial artery. In ancient Chinese texts, the blood flow and energy flow go together. Wherever blood flows, energy flows. The energy pulses, however, are not to be mistaken for the blood pulse. They are quite specific and distinct in themselves. There are twelve energy pulses, each one corresponding to a specific organ. The Traditional Acupuncture practitioner learns to feel the quantity and quality of each pulse, then to record it appropriately. The pulses are later correlated with the rest of the information from the examination. (See figure p. 114.)

The reading of the energy pulses is essential to diagnosis and treatment. A truly skilled practitioner can find in them the information of past illnesses, of present imbalances, and of future tendencies toward illness. Obviously this is a lifetime of learning.

> *The system of palpation propounded by the* Nei Ching *was believed to be effective in the nature and location of any kind of disease. The basis of this practice was the belief that the pulse actually consisted of six pulses, i.e., three sets of pulses on each hand, each connected with a particular part of the body and each able to record even the minutest pathological changes taking place within the body.*[2]

Each pulse is coupled with another, the Small Intestine with the Heart, the Gall Bladder with the Liver, the Bladder with the Kidney, the Large Intestine with the Lungs, the Stomach with the Spleen, and the Three Heater with Circulation Sex. The following quotes give a few examples of what can be felt in the pulses and what this might mean to a person's life.

> *The pulse is the storehouse of the blood. When the pulse beats are long and the strokes markedly prolonged, then the constitution of the pulse is well regulated; when the pulse beats are short and without volume, then the constitution of the pulse is out of order. When the pulse is quick, and contains six beats to one cycle of respiration, then it indicates heart trouble; and when the pulse is large the disease becomes grave.*[3]

> *When man is serene and healthy the pulse of the heart flows and connects, just as pearls are joined together or like a string of red jade—then one can speak of a healthy heart.*[4]

From the above descriptions, we start to understand what the pulses can tell us. Those descriptions are about one meridian, yet each has its own story, giving information about the state of the bodymind. Each of the pulses relates to an Element and to the correspondences of that Element. (See chapters on the Five Elements for detail.)

The chart of the Five Elements shows that the organs and functions are related to one another. The Heart, the Liver, the Kidneys, the Lungs, the Spleen, and Circulation Sex are often thought of as Yin functions. This is not correct since Yin never exists without Yang. It is more correct to say that these are the YINyang functions: the viscera, the sold mass organs, the storehouses. Their pulses are felt on the deep level of energy. On the superficial level are the yinYANG pulses: the Small Intestine, the Gall Bladder, the Bladder, the Large Intestine, the Stomach, and the Three Heater. The Chinese consider these to be the hollow organs, the bowels or workshop organs.

The Acupuncture practitioner holds the patient's right hand firmly and gently so that her arm is relaxed and easy. (The process described here is repeated on the patient's left hand.) Any obstruction like a watch, tight cuff or bracelet has to be removed. There are three pulse positions on each wrist, two levels of pulses at each position. The superficial level is felt by a very light palpation, and the deep level is felt with slightly more pressure. The method of pulsetaking never varies because this process requires absolute precision and accuracy. With her left hand, the Acupuncturist locates the pulse of the second position. This is the easiest one to find. (On the left hand it is the Gall Bladder pulse; on the right hand it is the Stomach pulse.) The other pulses are located relative to the second positions.

The first reading of the pulses is never the last in an examination or a treatment. They must be checked and re-checked to know the correctness and completeness of the reading and to make allowance for such variations as nervousness and anxiety. The practitioner's eyes are closed while taking pulses. This allows more concentrated focus of attention on each pulse and blocks out other distractions. Each pulse is recorded according to the norm established for that person. For example, we would not anticipate that a robust outdoor worker would have the same norm for her pulses as a sedate office worker. The norm is derived from each individual. There is not a Procrustean bed of pulses which everyone is made to fit. The pulse is recorded as a check if it feels normal, a plus ($+$) up to $3+$ if the pulse is hyper in volume, and a minus ($-$) up to minus 3 if the pulse is hypo in volume. The quantity of energy is the first quality that concerns us even though there are 27 other qualities on each pulse.

After the first pulse reading, the patient takes off all her clothing except underwear and lies on the table covered with a blanket. She may feel apprehensive, wondering what will happen, remembering media reports of people with dozens of needles stuck in them. Because most people have never experienced Traditional Acupuncture, I want to be sure and note that the examination is for gathering information from which we can determine if and how Acupuncture treatment can help. Until time is spent correlating the information from the exam, a diagnosis cannot be made. The needles and moxa are used during treatment and not before, except perhaps to be shown to an apprehensive patient at the end of the examination. Apprehension is usually relieved when a person sees that the needles are like filaments about the width of two hairs and not like hypodermics.

While the patient is lying down her pulses are taken again. At this point I usually ask a person to breathe deeply. This gives me a chance to see the depth of the breath and utilization of lung capacity. Breathing also helps relaxation. The patient is reminded that she can ask questions to find out what she wants to know. This freedom is important, especially since until then the practitioner has done all the asking. Often a person having treatment becomes quite articulate about Acupuncture in theory, as well as experientially. People are often curious and sometimes anxious to know what is happening with them. The descriptions and discussion about their pulses, their symptoms, the Elements and the Laws give the person a new language for health.

The next part of the examination is the abdominal diagnosis. We find the center pulse by placing the thumb and first three fingers over the umbilicus and pressing. This pulse should be in the center of the four fingers, which form a North-South, East-West axis. If it is off center in any direction it is massaged back into place to coincide with an energy pathway flowing straight up the center of the body. This meridian is called the Conception Vessel, a main source of the energy inherited from our parents. There are points on the Conception Vessel whose names give the spirit of this pathway: *Middle Palace, Great Deficiency, Sea of Ch'i (energy), Stone Gate.* The point at the umbilicus where the center pulse is, is called *Spirit Deficiency*. It is one of the points on the body forbidden to needle.

After finding the center pulse, specific areas of the abdomen are palpated. These areas correspond to the organ systems of the Meridians. Tenderness may indicate trouble in the Meridian. Along with this abdominal diagnosis, the alarm points are checked. These are special points of sensitivity. This information, too, says whether a Meridian is out of balance.

Next, the Three Chou are checked. These are divisions of the torso which correspond to the Three Heater. In the old texts these are called the *three burning spaces*. This function, little heeded in Western medicine, is analogous to the heating system in a house. When the temperature is even and comfortable, the occupants of the house carry on with their work in relative ease and harmony. If the temperature gets unbearably warm throughout, or even in part, the people living there are bound to feel concerned, upset, restless and unable to work. Likewise, if the house becomes unbearably cold in any part, the occupants react. The same is true in our bodies when the heating is not well regulated. These three areas tell us how the body is heating, whether there is harmony throughout the body and where there are places that are too hot or too cold. The Upper Chou is in the chest area. The two major organs within it are the Lungs and the Heart. The Middle Chou is above the umbilicus. The Liver, Gall Bladder, Spleen, Stomach and Small Intestine are within the Middle Chou. The Lower Chou is below the umbilicus and has within it the Bladder, the Kidneys and the Large Intestine. One could generally say that the Upper Chou controls respiration; the Middle, digestion and assimilation; and the Lower, elimination. The way we find out about the energy in the Three Heater is by feeling the areas. This is a developed sensitivity. We also know about the Three Heater via the pulses. You will remember that one of the Meridians within the Fire Element is the Three Heater. It commences at the nail of the third finger on the side adjacent to the little finger and ends at the lateral extremity of the eyebrow with 23 points. This means that we can affect the balance of that pathway of energy which controls the Three Chou by using any of the points along it. When a given symptom has not responded to any type of treatment, the reason is often because this function has not been considered in the entire picture of the patient. Heating of the emotional self, warmth and relationships with others are attributed to this Meridian and its sister, Circulation Sex. For this reason alone, we pay very special attention to this pathway, since it is often how we relate to other people that keeps us from being our healthy balanced selves.

Next we check the structure of the patient, that is, the vertebrae and the limbs and joints. A good chiropractor and osteopath are suggested to a person who needs a great deal of manipulative work, especially if she has never been thoroughly examined structurally. However, with the use of needles and moxa, the vertebrae can be realigned. It may take a bit longer than direct manipulation, but it is just as effective because it allows the muscles and tendons to relax before easing the bones back into place. Rotation or jamming of the cervical, thoracic or lumbar vertebrae affects the flow of energy in the bodymind. There is a major pathway called the Governor Vessel which travels up the center of the spinal column, up along the head to the front of the face where it meets the Conception

Vessel. The Bladder Meridian also runs in parallel lines along the spinal column. It has some special points that go directly to all the organs within the body. The relationship of structure and energy within the body is important. If the structure is aligned and sound, then the energy can flow the way it must, just as the people inside a house firmly built with correct, well-placed supports can move and interact freely without hindrance.

Just as any constriction in structure can cause a break in the energy flow, any block or constriction in musculature can also cause a break. Therefore, muscles are checked throughout the body for tone and blockage. Often, if the constriction is long standing, the muscle is actually knotted. If you have ever massaged the neck and shoulders of someone who carries tension there, you know what these knots feel like.

The body is continually telling us about ourselves. The Traditional Acupuncturist is taught to listen and take all the messages seriously. By saying this I do not mean to imply that other systems of healing do not also do this. I am not trying to impart an understanding of all therapies, but of Traditional Acupuncture.

The patient's pulses are read again. The time of day and season are recorded each time. Both of these make a slight but significant difference in the reading. For example, in winter, which is the season that corresponds to the Element Water, the pulses of the two Water functions, the Bladder and Kidneys, are expected to be a bit fuller than at any other time of year. The time of day is recorded for a similar reason based on the Chinese body clock. Each Meridian has its time of day for being just a bit fuller in energy. These are important variations that make a pulse reading absolutely accurate. Pulse-taking is used as the basis of diagnosis and working out of treatment and therefore *must* not be in error.

> *The Emperor said: I should like to be informed about the essential doctrines (of healing).*
>
> *Ch'i Po answered: The most important requirement of the art of healing is that no mistakes or neglect occur. There should be no doubt or confusion as to the application of the meaning of complexion and pulse. These are the maxims of the art of healing...*[5]

Another part of the examination is a procedure called Akabane. It is basically a Japanese method for verifying left-right imbalance within a Meridian. This imbalance can also be picked up in the pulses. The Akabane is a safeguard and the best way of finding an imbalance. It is essential to know that there is a left-right balance before any treatment. Before it can be in harmony with the other pathways, a Meridian must be balanced within itself.

How is Akabane done? A taper is lit and is passed equidistantly across a point at a constant height from that point. Each pass of the taper is counted and recorded. The left is standardly recorded over the right; for example, the Akabane of II (Small Intestine) is II L/R. The side with the greatest number of passes is the one deficient in energy. Though the flesh of the patient is not actually touched with the lighted taper, at a certain stage the point gets hot and the patient says *off*. The nail points of the pathways are used for this test. If the number of passes is not equal on both sides, then the first treatment that must be done is to balance the energy left-right.

In Traditional Acupuncture, the odour of a person is a diagnostic aid. I do not mean body odour, but rather a specific smell that corresponds to the imbalance of an Element. For example, the person with an imbalance in the Element Wood, that is the Liver and the Gall Bladder, is likely to have a rancid smell. This smell is usually not noticeable to the untrained nose and can be smelled only when a patient has her clothes off. However, it can be overwhelming, especially in chronic long-term diseases. Relating smells to illness is not a new phenomenon. Old-time Western physicians and Folk medicine knew the smell of many diseases.

Sounds are also diagnostically important to the Acupuncturist. We express in our voice the sound of our imbalance. A person with an imbalance in the Stomach and/or Spleen will likely have a singing sound in her voice, just as a person with an imbalance in the Lungs and/or Large Intestine would have a weeping sound. The ancient classic, *Nei Ching*, speaks about these connections:

> *Upon earth there is the transformation and change which produce the five flavors. The attainment of Tao (the Right Way) produces wisdom, while the supernatural (powers) spring from darkness and mystery.*

> *The supernatural (powers) create wind in Heaven and they create wood upon earth. Within the body they create muscles and of the five viscera they create the liver. Of the colors they create the green color and of the musical notes they create the note chio; and they give to the human voice the ability to form a shouting sound...* [6]

Like sounds, emotions are also important diagnostically. A person's description of herself emotionally is an important part of the examination. *Anger is injurious to the liver, but sympathy counteracts anger.*

If a person has difficulty or feels stuck in any one emotion, she is asking for help for the energy that feeds the organs most related to that emotion.

During the examination the Acupuncture practitioner feels the pathways as they traverse the body bilaterally. Often a Meridian feels cold in the area of blockage. It may also feel void in certain places and hot in others. These differences are often barely perceptible, but the information they give is valuable for diagnosis. Skin texture changes, temperature, colorations, bruises and scars may be further evidence of imbalance in a pathway.

The tongue is examined for texture and coloration. It is divided into areas that correspond to the Elements.

There is also a method of diagnosis that deals with the iris of the eye. It is often used for adjunct information in the Acupuncture examination. The iris is divided into specific areas that correspond to organs and functions within the human being. By studying the eye, one can cross-check information derived elsewhere from the body. The clarity of the eyes and how a person makes eye contact are important in Traditional Acupuncture diagnosis.

The pulses are read again. This is the last thing to be done in the examination. It is a final check on the earlier pulse findings. The chapter on treatment following this chapter on examination gives more information on how the pulses are used.

The entire examination is a lengthy process involving the whole person. What I have presented to you is a maximum outline. The actual flow of the exam varies from person to person. One patient may have a facility to express herself in response to the questions; another may be reticent or shy; another untrusting, suspicious; another loquacious. There are as many examinations as there are people, so that the style and experience of one exam may only vaguely resemble the next. For example, an African man, during the verbal part of the examination, never sat down for longer than a minute. He was gesticulating, stalking around the room, questioning me, and answering questions like the one on age with *I'm twenty floods ago.*

The traditional diagnosis process respects the integrity and individuality of each person. There is no correct way to answer, or judgement made on the different information that comes up during an examination. It is not a test or a contest. There is no grade. The only thing necessary is to see, to hear, to ask, and to feel what the bodymind of the person is saying. And though we usually allow about two hours for the entire examination, it may take more or less time. Another variable in the examination process is the expertise of the practitioner. For example, Dr. Worsley, who is my teacher and who has been practicing for twenty-seven years, does a thorough examination in a much shorter time. However, the information we gather is the same even though he goes about it differently. His mastery of pulse reading gained over the years enables him to rely much more on the pulses without needing as many of the other cross-checking diagnostic aids.

As you can see from the outline of the examination, questions are asked that are intimate to a person's life. The depth and breadth of the examination ask a person to stretch beyond her usual thought processes. Some people have trouble doing this. The Acupuncturist can help by rewording, giving examples and going slowly enough to allow a person the space she needs to respond. In itself the examination can and often does act as an opening to the healing process by giving a person the chance to gather together disparate aspects of her life.

Chapter Eight

Traditional Diagnosis and Treatment

Traditional Diagnosis

This section will explain how the diagnosis is done.[1] All the information about the health of a person that has been gathered in the examination is looked at in the light of the Five Elements and their correspondences. Each bit of information says something about at least one of the Elements. These messages may be like notices on a bulletin board calling attention to something that's happening, or about to happen; they may be a sign of serious alarm, or signaling a long-term distress. Whatever the information is saying, it refers to the Ch'i Energy and therefore must be noticed. By pulling this together, like gathering wild flowers into a bouquet, we can see the entirety of a person's life and know how or if health can be restored by Acupuncture treatment. This discernment of the state of the Ch'i Energy is the diagnosis of a person's health. The description of the diagnosis is given in terms of the Elements. Once the diagnosis is made treatment can begin.

The following is part of an examination. It is an illustration of the process of diagnosis: Mary is 56 years old, born April 11, 1917 in the morning around 9:00 A.M. She runs a shop and is on her feet a lot. She is a big woman with bumpy *goose* flesh and mottled skin. She is wearing a blue and yellow dress. She came to have Acupuncture treatment because: *I have a pain in my right hip and thigh, a gnawing like an ache. It's there all the time. It feels hot and nothing helps it. About seven years ago when I worked in a museum I was sitting in a chair in a nylon overall. The chair was slippery and I fell off it onto my tail. It started to ache and became more and more painful, a shocking sharp pain. I suffered it. I didn't tell anyone. I'm like that; I'm afraid. I was put into a plaster cast but was allergic to it and became worse. I was nearly demented. I have a history of swollen feet and I fall over a lot. My hands and feet are always cold. I have a weakness in my heart. I had scarlet fever at age three. I worry about people, others, not myself. I'm a terrible worrier. I can't just sit still, I've got to be doing something. I am chronically constipated, sometimes only one motion a week. I sometimes get very depressed and I feel I could do something desperate. My first husband tried to commit suicide and has been a missing person for years now. I love the husband I have now. I took care of my mother til she died from heart trouble at age 80. (She began to cry and I took her hand.) I started to put on weight after a hysterectomy 15 years ago. I have a recurring dream that I am too heavy and cannot get up. I had one child, a son, 26 years ago. It was a hard birth . . . he weighed 12½ lbs. He has a skin problem due to nervousness. I love sweet things. I am fond of pork. I have lost confidence in myself. I detest winter, especially after Christmas, and I love the spring. I bruise easily. Yellow is my favorite color. People think I'm a 'good-hearted soul.'*

In Mary's pulses the biggest imbalances are in Water and Earth. The Spleen and Stomach pulse both read +2, which means an excess in energy or hyperfunctioning. The Bladder and Kidney pulse both read −2, which means a deficiency in Energy or hypo-functioning. The Fire pulses, especially Circulation Sex and Three Heater, are also deficient in Energy, but less so than the Water pulses.

Though the above is not the entire examination, it is a complete enough excerpt to illustrate how the messages are interpreted to make a diagnosis about the state of Mary's Ch'i energy. This is done in terms of the Elements. The diagnosis: Mary's Earth Element is in most distress. The predominant emotion in her life is sympathy, with a history of compassion toward others even at the expense of her own well being. Her connection with the earth beneath her feet is not very stable as she described in her *falling over* off the chair. As she walks it is relatively easy to see her disconnection and listing to one side. A history of swollen ankles is significant in relation to earth . . . feet are our bodily contact point with the ground and the force of gravity. For Mary this contact is not clear and firm. The two Earth pulses are the Stomach and Spleen. Both of them are excessive in volume—the Earth is trying desperately hard to do its work but to little avail. This manifests itself in Mary's life via the pain in her hip and thigh. Her excessive weight and dreams of being *too heavy and cannot get up* cry out the Earth imbalance. The things that carry her weight are her legs. In Chinese concepts the hips and thighs are associated most often with the Spleen, a function within the Earth Element. Yellow is her favorite color, and it is the color correspondence of Earth. Flesh is governed by the Element Earth, and hers is goose bumply. It is not a smooth clean expanse. She is fidgety . . . *I can't sit still.* The function of the Spleen is the transporter or distributor. From her cold hands and feet as well as her uneasiness in body, it is clear that distribution of energy is not happening as it is needed. Think of the body as a kingdom: there are parts of her kingdom where the transportation system is not functioning, especially the outlying districts and the extremities. These are cut off from the main flow of activity, even though they are so important to the workings of the entire kingdom.

The Stomach has the function of nourishing, rotting and ripening the food, assimilating and bringing to fruition all that one takes in. Though she is overweight, Mary is not being nourished nearly enough by her diet, which includes lots of sweets. This is significant. Her favorite taste is sweet. This reiterates the Earth imbalance going on in the Ch'i Energy. Her chronic constipation is partly coming from the hard attempts of the Earth to do what it needs to. She cannot budge on the inside, even though in other ways she cannot stay still. Now, it is also clear in the examination that many signals point to distress within the Water Element. The symptom of constipation speaks of lack of lubrication, the fluidity within the elimination process. Her swollen ankles are a result of blockage in Water creating soggy Earth which cannot hold anything upright very well, and which creates a lack of confidence in one's own ability to stand up straight. The pain and ache in Mary's hip come from the stress upon her system to have fluidity of motion. Her Earth is too firm and hard in some places and soggy weak in others. Her voice sings.

Now, even though all that I have said is true of the symptoms Mary expresses, the cause of the imbalance in Earth and in Water is in the Element Fire. When she was three Mary had scarlet fever. To the Chinese this is considered the *fire of fire* fevers. Fifty-three years ago this imbalance happened within the Energy and was never righted. Even though the Earth Element, the child of Fire, is the one hollering, there are signs from Fire that it is in trouble. Mary bruises easily, she says she has a *weakness in my heart*, and people think of her as a *good-hearted soul.* Her Fire pulses are deficient in Energy . . . alarmingly so, especially in the functions of Circulation Sex and Three Heater, but also in the Heart. The relationships she has had in her life have been very difficult with her husband, her ailing mother, and even with her 26-year-old son; she has always given warmth and affection and always yearned for it to be given to her. Her own Energy is depleted here. Circulation Sex, the Protector of the Supreme Controller the Heart, has been taking all the blows in order to keep the Controller functioning properly. In the process of doing this the Protector has taken a beating. It is weak. The pulse is a − 2. Mary's natural body defenses are very stressed, and so she eats for nourishment and strength. Her fat is a form of protection in place of her innate strength, but it only drains her of energy because with it she has to carry around more stress.

Fire is the causative factor of Mary's symptoms; therefore, the treatments will be directed toward rebalancing the energy in the Fire Element.

For each patient this gathering of information is done. The description of the Elements as they are within an individual patient is based on the information from the examination. Every diagnosis is unique, because every person is unique and has her own life's combination of messages.

Treatment

Once the diagnosis is made the treatment can begin. What is an Acupuncture treatment? How does it work? What is happening to the patient? How do we go about choosing the points to use? What is a point? This section describes the treatment process. Real life situations illustrate what happens, the patient's response and my own involvement and perspective.

Illness is an imbalance of the Energy within us. Examination involves listening to the bodymind tell us where to find that imbalance. Treatment is restoration of the balance, moving the Energy where it needs to go so that the healing process can happen and health returns.

> *The Emperor exclaimed: Very well! and then he said: To treat and to cure disease means to examine the body, the breath, the complexion, its glossiness or degree of moisture and the pulse, as to whether it is flourishing or deteriorating, and whether the disease is a recent one. But then the actual treatment must follow, for later on there is no time.*[2]

> *By inserting needles (Acupuncture) or burning small cones of punk (moxibustion) at these sites the doctor attempts by his interference to restore proper phasing of the energetic flow, to restore it to that dynamic balance in the order of time which for Chinese defines health.*[3]

Treatment itself is akin to a system of gates and doors; a good image is the system of locks and gates of a waterway. The needle acts as the opener or closer of those gates and doors, summoning, allowing, pushing, pulling the energy to and from one pathway to another. This is done via individul points along a pathway. It *does* make a difference whether the point is actually found. If it is not, then the pulse change will not occur. The pulses, at this stage, are the Acupuncturist's greatest guide as to whether or not the energy can move and is moving.

Let us say that I wish to move energy from the Gall Bladder Meridian to the Small Intestine. I choose the Wood point of the Small Intestines and with a needle manipulation summon the energy from the Gall Bladder to the Small Intestines. The volume of energy in the Small Intestines should increase, and the volume of energy in the Gall Bladder should decrease. If there is no change, I must ask whether or not I hit the point and whether or not the energy can move. A chronic blockage in energy will take several treatments before the pulse change begins to hold firmly.

The number of needles in any one treatment varies, but basically follows the law of least action. This states that the fewer the number of needles used to affect the desired change, the better.

The energy flows in a clockwise direction, and the balancing of it by transferring and summoning from one place to another follows the same flow. The Law of the Five Elements, as discussed in chapter one, describes the movement of energy. Each Element is nourished by the one preceding it and nourishes the one following it. This is known as the Shen cycle, the creative movement of energy. Within this cycle there are other laws: the Law of Parent-Child (also known as the Law of Mother-Son) describes the special nourishing role within the Five Elements. Dr. Worsley uses the following example for illustration: a nursing mother who is strong, healthy and happy provides a full flow of nourishment for her child. What happens if the mother gets upset, doesn't feel well, or is not being fed well herself? The quality of milk suffers and probably the amount. This in turn causes the child to cry from hunger and undernourishment, even though it is the mother who is in trouble and needs help. This same thing is true with the Elements. The mother Element may be the one needing attention, even though it is the child who is hollering the most. This illustrates the folly of treating symptoms. They may be doing the hollering, but they are not the cause. If we say to a child *it's okay* and slip her a piece of candy to quiet her when she hollers, we may get a few moments rest, but she will only cry louder when she realizes she is not getting what she needs. In the meantime, the mother is still wanting help.

If a person comes in for Acupuncture complaining of symptoms like pains and tightness in the chest, pains down the arm, especially on the left side, shortness of breath, one of the first suspicions that might cross a practitioner's mind would be trouble in the Heart. The hollering is being done by the Heart, but what is the cause? In the course of examination, we may find that the Wood Element is imbalanced and therefore cannot feed Fire, thus symptoms come from Fire. This does not mean that trouble in Fire is always coming from Wood, but it does mean that we must be very sure to know what is happening among all the Elements in order to find the cause of imbalance. Once we find the cause, we can then put right the energy according to the Laws, and thus the symptoms will disappear.

Another part of the Law of Parent-Child (Mother-Son) is the possibility that the son is the cause of the symptoms that arise in the mother. For example, an unruly obstreperous child who demands every moment of the mother's attention, giving her not a moment's rest, may result in a frantic parent tearing out her hair and feeling unable to cope. In this instance the cries go out from the parent while the cause rests with the child who is draining the mother. Now obviously, things are never as clear-cut as this, because there is so much interaction and interresponsibility, but it is possible to alter the situation by helping the main culprit begin to feel better. If we look at the Law of Mother-Son in terms of Nature, we see that this relationship is continuously happening. Wood feeds Fire. If the Wood is too dry, the Fire will rage and so on.

The constant interaction among the Elements is what keeps us healthy, provided that each of the Elements and the functions within it are balanced. If one Element is out of harmony, it is not long before the rest begin to feel the effects and go off balance. It is up to the skill of the Acupuncturist to decide where the treatment will begin in order to put the entire system on the road to health.

The Energy flows in a continuous circuit along specific pathways. Where to begin balancing is only known through the traditional diagnosis. Points are chosen on the basis of all the considerations for moving Energy, and all of these considerations follow the natural laws as described in the Five Elements. Within any one treatment, it is possible to move the Energy, but it must always be done with the awareness of the entire bodymind of a person so that too much is not asked at one time. The process of healing must be organic. The names and spirits of the points are also important in deciding on a specific treatment pattern.

Another aspect of the Five Elements is the K'o cycle, a control cyle of Energy. Remember that unless each Element is kept within bounds, it could become off balance. This cycle can be thought of as the forces that keep the planets in their orbits. Furthermore, the destructive disease called aggressive energy travels across this cycle. If it reaches three Elements, then a person is beyond help and will surely die soon. If two Elements are affected, the person is gravely ill and may not be able to be helped. Aggressive energy has to be drained out of the body. If it is allowed to remain, the person's life is in danger because once one Element is affected, another will follow unless this aggressive energy is removed. The draining is done via specific Acupuncture points with a manipulation used only for draining aggressive energy. These points are on the back. If Acupuncture treatment is carried out on a person without first draining the aggressive energy, the practitioner runs the risk of spreading this destructive force throughout the body. If for no other reason than this, one can see the need for the Acupuncturist to be a highly skilled person.

Another law within the Five Elements is the law of balance *within* each meridian. Since the 12 main meridians are all bilateral, it is important to know that there is harmony within the pathway itself, and that there is not a discrepancy in the volume of energy on either side of the meridian. If there is an imbalance within a pathway, the first treatment will attend to this rebalance. A pathway of energy pulling against itself can only cause chaos and confusion in the bodymind.

Acupuncture treatment attends to these and all the other laws that govern the movement of Ch'i Energy. Acupuncture treatment is done with needles and with an herb called *moxa*. A needle is inserted into an Acupuncture point along a meridian in order to move the flow of energy in the direction of balance and harmony. Because this energy is the Life Force within us, as it is summoned and directed via the needles, it will cause changes that can be felt. Sometimes at the insertion of a needle, a patient will experience a sensation of flow in a part of their body. Sometimes there is no noticeable feeling, not even awareness that a needle has been inserted. Between treatments is usually when a person notices that something different and inexplicable is happening within them. Because Traditional Acupuncture deals with the whole person in bodymind-spirit, the experience of changes may occur on any level of human experience and usually on all levels during the course of treatment.

The needles are of the finest quality stainless steel, though down through the ages they have been made of flint and of varieties of metal, including gold and silver. Because of a sudden Western interest in Acupuncture, there is at present a proliferation of needle types. The best are master needles—the simplest and most finely made. They are durable, strong and fine. Thickness varies, but the needle commonly used is about two or three hairs width, like a filament, not like a hypodermic. The length also varies, but the most common lengths are one-half inch and one inch for the needle itself, though the shaft is considerably longer since it is used for holding the needle and directing the insertion into the Acupuncture point. There are many different manipulations and needle techniques.

The needle for acupuncture must be applied quietly and with utmost care.[4]

The herb *moxa*, or artemisia vulgaris latiflora, has been known for centuries. It has healing properties within it. In Traditional Acupuncture moxa is used in many ways, all of which involve burning. It is rolled into tiny cones which are placed one at a time on an Acupuncture point and lit. It is left on the point until it gets hot, and then it is removed so as not to burn the patient. In some countries the tradition is to leave the moxa on the skin until it burns all the way down, producing a blister and a long-lasting scar. Leaving it on makes very little difference in effect and would be unthinkable in a Western culture. I have seen people in other cultures proudly displaying their moxa burns in the same way an old scar might cause excitement and fascination. I cannot imagine people in the United States proudly showing off their moxa burns.

Moxa on an Acupuncture point brings changes in the energy in a way similar to those produced by the needle when it is used as described above. It can be placed over a thin slice of ginger to avoid the danger of burning a patient, yet still retains its beneficial effect on the Energy.

Another way of using moxa is to wrap it around the shaft of the needle, after the needle is inserted, and then to light it. This is often used on Acupuncture points around joints that have articulation and mobility trouble. A ball of moxa is placed on the end of the needle and lit until it all burns. This warms the area, and though the actual needle does not get hot, the heat and the healing effect are transmitted to the point. This helps to alter severe Energy blockages. Another way moxa is used is to roll it into a thick stick. This is for warming areas of the body like the neck and shoulders, where muscles are often tight and unrelaxed. Passing the roll over the area is soothing and warming. This type of moxa is sometimes used for acne problems if a person's face is able to stand the heat. It draws the toxicity out of the body.

There are many different needle manipulations and techniques to move the Energy. In speaking of this the ancient classic says: *one must first feel with the hand and trace the system of the body . . . on the outside one should treat the openings which are left by the needle so that they close up and so that the spirit can remain within. When all the breath is spent at the exhalation, one should insert the needle and wait for some time until the patient has to inhale, as though one waited for something precious, and were unconscious of day and night. When the breath is entirely exhausted in exhalation, one should move the needle, but with great care and caution.*[5] This quote describes the process of one form of needle manipulation. There are several others, and each is specific and done with as great a care as described in the quote. It is, after all, via the needle that the change in the energy is brought about. A practitioner can feel whether or not she is on the Acupuncture point and whether the energy is being moved via the needle. The pulse changes verify the movement of Energy.

The practitioner of Traditional Acupuncture must be expertly trained and infinitely dedicated. Helping sick people to get well takes tremendous clarity, and therefore the health of the practitioner is important. The balance needed to clearly see the process of health and illness in oneself is the same balance needed to be able to see the process in another. This does not mean that the Acupuncturist is superhumanly healthy, or unsusceptible to illness. It means that she has experienced the workings of her bodymind under treatment and also knows the feel of the needles and moxa. This gives her an awareness of the anxiety that some patients have toward needles. It also maintains her own health. *Those who are habitually without disease help to train and to adjust those who are sick, for those who treat should be free from illness. By observing myself I know about others and their diseases are revealed to me, and by observing external symptoms one gathers knowledge about internal disturbances.*[6] Other excerpts from the ancient classic ask us to bear in mind the consequence of bad Acupuncture. *Poor medical workmanship is neglectful and careless and must be therefore combatted, because a disease that is not completely cured can easily breed new disease or there can be a relapse of the old disease.*[7] *... if a physician reverses and spoils the natural condition of a body, health can never again be recovered.*[8]

These are not easy words. If the Life Force within us is to be treated, the physician to whom we turn for help must be more than competent in the workings of the body. She must be true to the Life Force within herself and sure that what she does with the Life Force of another is done with the knowledge and integrity that respect another's Life Energy.

Traditional Acupuncture *is* a powerful medicine. It can do good things to help people, but in unscrupulous hands it can be misleading. One of the bad things it can do is to give to sick people the false impression that Acupuncture can cure everything for everybody all the time and do it quickly. This is bad because it promotes the idea that Acupuncture is either a cure-all for everyone or a process like a Band-Aid or an aspirin for symptoms, with nothing else to say to a human being.

The classical writings often made reference to life style and how this affects our internal and external balance. If we look at Nature throughout a cycle of seasons, we can observe an order with only occasional excess. The philosophy of Tao is one of harmony, not of extremity, and so the way a person leads her own life follows the same guide of harmony if she is trying to live in accord with herself. *Nowadays people are not like this; they use wine as beverage and they adopt recklessness as usual behavior. They enter the chamber (of love) in an intoxicated condition; their passions exhaust their vital forces; their cravings dissipate their true (essence); they do not know how to find contentment within themselves; they are not skilled in the control of their spirits. They devote all their attention to the amusement of their minds, thus cutting themselves off from the joys of long (life). For this reason they reach only one half of the hundred years and then they degenerate.*[9] This quote describes the lifestyle that is habitually in excess, not the lifestyle of occasional binges. Yet, in its essence the description comes very close to the symptoms of malaise imbedded in present day life. So when I talk about the person who is ill and her involvement in restoring herself to health with the help of Acupuncture, I refer also to the living of a wise and healthful life whose excitement is in harmony, not in excess.

Even though Acupuncture can and does work on people who are skeptical, or who do not clearly want to get better, the whole process is more beneficial if the patient is cooperating in her own health and well-being. It is true in any healing profession that the person who wants health and works to get better, who does not leave everything up to the physician, is far more likely to be healthy. In the *Nei Ching* Ch'i Po says to the Yellow Emperor: *This is the way of Acupuncture: if man's vitality and energy do not propel his own will his disease cannot be cured.*[10] *Once the spirit has turned away it will as a rule not return.*[11] *It is difficult to cure one who is bound to die.*[12]

Along with the concept of health is the awareness of death. Balance and harmony does not mean never dying. Death is ever present, even though the exact personal moment cannot be ascertained. The preparation we make for death is the same that we make for health, and for life. The key to health and to life is consciousness, being as much of ourselves as we can be at any given moment, being whole and harmonized internally, being at one with the world externally. Once we begin to realize that the Life Force energizing us individually is the same Life Force uniting us, and that the Energy never dies, the prospect of death takes on a dignity and a promise. Acupuncture, though it may not be able to alleviate the cause of everyone's symptoms, can offer the possibility of learning about energy and consciousness on a personal, very intimate level. As a tool we can use it to bring ourselves to the balance that is possible even as death waits close by. We can learn to live in integrity and harmony within and without. We can learn to die the same way.

A course of treatment varies from individual to individual. Generally one would have a month of treatment for every year of illness. That is a very rough guide and usually it takes less time, but the bodymindspirit needs time to harmonize within itself. If we understood the process toward illness, we would certainly better understand the process toward health. The one-needle *cures* often seen in the media are usually quick temporary removal of a symptom without getting to its cause. Traditional Chinese Acupuncture is *not* palliation or suppression of symptoms. It is all involvement with the innate workings of a person in bodymindspirit to remove the cause of the symptom. This cannot be said often enough.

The Acupuncturist knows whether Acupuncture can help a person by assessing what needs doing via the diagnosis and feeling whether the Ch'i Energy can and will move. Once the Energy begins to be balanced, the changes can be felt on the pulses. The patient can also feel the changes in herself, her life and her symptoms. There is rarely a case where Traditional Acupuncture cannot do some amount of rebalancing which will enable a person to feel better in herself, even though her symptoms may not alter significantly. In this healing art, feeling good in oneself, one's very center, is a very important sign of health.

Chapter Nine

A Case Report

A Case Report

The Traditional Acupuncture Examination is a loving walk into the life of another; into the field of wild flowers uniquely this person, gathering the bouquet, seeing the colors, smelling the fragrances, touching the petals and leaves, observing the arrangement, listening to the sounds and silences, inquiring sensuously (via the senses) into the nature of this particular person, this incomparable constellation of life's phenomena, life's showings. Our person is Mike.

Distinctions for Listening

In being with Mike, as with any person who asks me to be their practitioner, I am called to listen to life as it lives through them, to listen without conclusions, even when they have concluded themselves. For example, with Mike, when he says "I am the kind of person that likes to be alone," I can hear that he has made a conclusion that disallows other possibilities. We, as human beings, do this all the time. The question is, is there an observer present to make the distinction between conclusions and phenomena? That Mike is alive is the phenomenon. Whatever else he or we may say about that is a conclusion or story. And in our conclusions, in our stories, is where unnecessary suffering resides. What Mike says about life will determine his peacefulness and possibility. My work is to listen and assist him to reveal the distinction between phenomenon and conclusion. My offering is to be an observer, so that he can open some new conversations big enough to live in, big enough for those who journey through life with Mike to live in. Because we are human and because as human beings we speak and listen, we will continue to make stories, draw conclusions, create conversations. To observe that, to reveal our conclusions, then to construct new and larger conversations is integral to the art of healing, the art of being alive.

The following is the text of Mike's life as he has it storied—this includes my inquiry, and a mixture of the phenomena with the stories he has about the phenomena: what we usually call a "history." These are Mike's own words. One of my intentions in being with Mike, or any of my patients, is for him to recognize himself as an observer of his own life. Observing phenomena, he becomes a learner in the daily dance of creation, enabling him to create new and more live-able conversations.

> **Give a person a fish, they eat for a day.**
> **Teach a person to fish and they eat for a lifetime.**

Name: Mike

Physical Description: 5 ft. 11 in. tall, 165 lbs. He enters wearing baggy jeans, a blue t-shirt, boots, a heavy jacket and glasses. He is clean shaven with short dark hair. Mike's nails are bitten down to the quick. I am struck immediately by his affable demeanor. He appears eager and open. He smiles easily and frequently.

Age: 21

Date of Birth: 10-1-72

Marital Status: single

Children: none

Occupation: recent college graduate

Welcome. I'm Dianne. I'm happy to be with you. Shall I call you Mike?
Yes, that's what my friends and family call me. (He smiles, warm and open.)

Mike, shall we begin the inquiry into this work we are about to do together? Can we start with a few basic questions?
That sounds good to me. (His voice is deep and serious.)

Do you have a favorite season?
I really like them all, though I prefer the autumn —all the changes and colors of the trees.... I don't much like the mud in the springtime.

What is your favorite color?
I like bright colors. All the primary colors. I'm maybe a bit partial to blue.

Is there a time of day you like best?
I really like early morning—6 a.m. I love to see the sunrise and sunset— the dawn and dusk.

If you had to pick a favorite place in nature, what would it be?
It's a toss-up between the ocean and the forest—Muir Woods takes my breath away.

What is your favorite taste?
I love spicy, very hot food—curry, Cajun, Szechuan. I like sweets a lot, too. I really like all different tastes.

What is your relationship to food?
I love it! Eating is one of my favorite pastimes. I love tasting and experimenting with all kinds of things. I like to cook, too. I do worry about my weight though, so I work out a lot. I think I could get very fat, if I let myself go. My dad is kind of overweight.

How is your vision?
I'm nearsighted without my eyeglasses. I couldn't see the chalk board when I was younger [about 7 years old]. I've tried contacts but my eyes don't seem to like them.

And your hearing?
My hearing is good. Sometimes my sense of hearing seems very acute, like when I'm in the woods listening to birds. I'm a good bird caller.

How are your teeth?
My teeth are strong and straight—I didn't have to have braces when I was a kid. I don't have a single cavity. My teeth are the talk of the family!

What is your skin like?
In hot weather I get these rashes on my chest and back. They itch. I sometimes get them after exercise, too.

How is your sense of smell?
I think my smeller isn't so great. My mom always says to stop and smell the flowers. The fragrance of roses is wasted on me.

What is breathing like for you, Mike?
Part of why I'm here is asthma. I had pneumonia when I was 8. I like to exercise, but I have to be very careful or I end up not being able to breathe. (His color changes here—red to white. His voice goes lower—the sound of weeping. He gets very serious. Later on, when we speak more about asthma his demeanor also changes.)

What is your relationship to sleep?
I'm a sound sleeper. I snore a lot, too. Or so they tell me. It runs in my family, I guess. My father snores and so does my mother! (Laughs) When I sleep on my stomach or my side it's not so bad.

And dreaming?
I want to remember my dreams more. That was something I was

thinking about asking—if acupuncture helps with remembering dreams. I'd like to remember the ones that aren't nightmares. I remember those pretty clearly, usually.

How are your bowels?
Regular, every morning. I don't usually think about it, although I did get a bit constipated when I first started the medicine.

What medications do you take?
I started taking cortisone for the asthma a year ago, and whatever stuff is in the inhaler.

How is your urination?
Fine.

What is your digestion like?
I'm good here! Occasionally I get heart-burn, if I eat really hot stuff on an empty stomach.

Perspiration?
I sweat a lot in the summer. My feet get really hot. I have to sleep with them outside the covers. Sometimes in the summer I sleep with wet washcloths on my feet to cool them off!

How is your circulation?
I tend to be pretty warm, in general. That's why I like the autumn and winter and don't like the summer so much.

What is your relationship to alcohol and drugs?
I used to smoke pot occasionally. I found it very relaxing, and there are certain friends I enjoyed smoking with. Now, with the asthma, I need to pay attention to my body. I liked the marijuana. I'm sorry to give it up... I don't drink much, but when I do I love either scotch or a tequila drink—all the better if I can mix it with something like lime juice.

What about beverages?
I don't like coffee. I drink tea. I love sour drinks. In the summer I drink a lot of limeade. I make concoctions in the blender with all kinds of different juices.

Do you smoke?
No. I tried cigarettes a few times with friends and never liked it. I couldn't inhale without embarrassing myself.

With whom do you live, Mike?

With my mom and dad and my sister Janie. She's 13. We live here in town. I graduated from college last semester and now I'm looking for a job. Then I'll get a place of my own.

What prompted you to come for acupuncture treatment? What did you hear? Who spoke with you about it?
In the gym one day my friend Mark heard me wheezing and breathing really hard, and saw me using an inhaler. A year ago the doctor had told me I have asthma—"adult onset" or something like that. Mark knows you. His mom gets acupuncture, so he told me I should check it out. I hate it when I can't breathe. I get mad and it scares me. I'm too young to be sick. Anyway, it's not the only thing that bugs me. (His voice goes very low here.)

What else are you bugged about, Mike?
I have a whole list. I did okay in college, but I still don't know what I really want to do. I have nightmares sometimes that wake me up; someone is chasing me and I get lost trying to escape. And it seems like I'm tired a lot. I can get really down on myself. (His face flushes a bit here.)

Anything else?
Yes, but I wasn't going to say anything. My steady girlfriend, Cathy, just left for grad school. She wants to be free to date other guys, and we hadn't been doing too well. She finally told me sex with me wasn't very satisfying. I know what she means. My orgasm comes pretty fast, I guess. It makes me upset. It puts tension in our relationship. I don't know what to do. I don't know if acupuncture can help with something like this. Can it? (His color is blue here. The sound is low and groaning. The emotion is fear.)

I don't know yet, Mike. Let me keep listening as you tell me more about yourself. I'm beginning to hear some connections in what you're telling me. It is clear that your "squawks," that is to say, your symptoms, are asking you to pay attention to life in some significant ways. I use the word squawk not to diminish the symptom, but to avoid a label that would make you a person with a disease rather than a person with an embodied living call from life. Tell me your mood and what you say about life. Even though it may sound awkward, tell me who you say you are.
My grandmother comes to mind when you ask me this. She was my dad's mother. We were really close. She always told me that life was about us all loving each other. I like that idea. It makes me feel better when I think like that. A lot of what I think about myself comes from her. Like I feel that I have a good heart. I care about people—especially

my family and friends and Cathy. (His voice rises and falls; singing.) My grandmother always told me I am very compassionate. I think I also could stand to be more disciplined. I tried to study hard in school and college and I did pretty well. But maybe not as well as I should have. (Easy and smiling again, yet somewhat uncertain.)

Tell me more about your grandmother.
My sister and I spent a lot of time at her house growing up. We would hang out there a lot, especially when my mom wasn't feeling well or was tired. My sister was a baby at the time. My grandmother told a lot of stories. And she read to me. Even after I knew how to read I used to like for her to read to me. And there were a lot of kids in the neighborhood where she lived. We'd play Capture the Flag until it got so dark outside we couldn't see and we'd have to come in. She didn't mind if we built forts in her back yard or had water-balloon fights—so long as we didn't track water into the house or get too carried away. She would sing to me, too. We would sing together. She taught me lots of songs... oldies that I still know! I loved going to her house. She died a year and a half ago... from a heart attack. I miss her. I could talk about everything with her, even sex. She was really the only one I did talk to. (His voice is hollow here—grief.)

Mike, though I am not your wonderful grandmother, will you talk to me about sex so I can hear how you think about it?
I am a little embarrassed. It seems so unmanly to have any trouble with sex, and I don't hear any of my friends or other guys talking about having this experience. And to talk about it with you—you're a woman and all. But then so was my grandma and so is Cathy. It's not so easy to trust. I just couldn't stand to be laughed at. I'm kind of old-fashioned even though I started learning about sex very young, about 7 years old. My family is Catholic and sex was a sin except if you were married to make babies. I got confused and I didn't have anybody to talk to. I guess most kids don't. It was always a secret and something to get over with fast so as not to get caught doing something bad.... I just realized something, I still do that! (He gets quite excited here—genuinely making a connection he hadn't had before. It is a wonderful little moment, an "aha!")

Who is Cathy for you?
Well, she has a great sense of humor. It's fun to be around her. She's also pretty serious, though. I mean she has very strong emotions. She doesn't always share them with other people, not even me. She kind of covers them up with humor. But then something will happen and she'll finally end up saying what's really going on for her. That's how it happened that she ended up telling me about wanting to see other

guys... I think she was happy with me before, though, when we first started going out. That was part of what I liked about her so much—how much she seemed to really genuinely like me! It made me feel really good to be with her. She's also really pretty... (He reddens.)

What are you learning now, Mike?
What do you mean?

What might it be possible for you to learn from this upset about how much intimacy with a woman means to you. Maybe this is an opportunity to learn some new ways of being... maybe more sensual, less sexual, or less genital-sexual. Maybe, even though, as you say, you have had sexual experiences since a young age, maybe you could declare yourself a beginner at sex?
A beginner? That doesn't seem so great. I mean the whole thing has been about getting experience...

Being a beginner could give you some freedom with sex—some chance to play! To make it all new, all for the first time. Letting go of this conversation of "I feel guilty and this needs to be over quickly." There's nothing wrong with that as a conversation—maybe there's just no freedom in it, no room to breathe. What do you say about that?
I don't know what to say. I have been thinking there is no hope for me with this, and even feeling like "so what, it doesn't really matter anyway." When you said no room to breathe that got my attention. What if all this is connected? I sure feel like a rookie—what did you call it, a beginner? Maybe if I just lighten up, I'll start to feel better. (He looks like a light just went on!)

Mike, you said that a doctor told you that you have asthma. Tell me, what does that mean to you? What was happening physically that you went to the doctor? What was happening in your life then?
I was beginning my senior year in college. I had spent my junior year in Italy and was returning to ordinary school. Cathy was questioning being my girlfriend. Graduation was getting closer. I didn't know what to do with a poli-sci degree. I felt I couldn't breathe, and then physically I really couldn't breathe. My chest got so tight, closed down, and I panicked. Nothing like that had ever happened to me before. I had always taken breathing for granted. Not any more. I thought I could count on my body—now I'm not certain anymore. In fact I'm not certain about anything. It's pretty scary. It makes me anxious about the future. I wheeze and get an attack of this stuff pretty often, especially with exertion. (He is very solemn here; color ashen, sound weeping. This is unlike most of the rest of the time when red, the sound of laughter, and an affable smiling demeanor show.)

How come you call it an attack? Could you think about it any other way?

It comes on like something hitting me. I did think at first that it was my heart since my chest gets so tight. I was glad it wasn't! And, I'm lucky it's not cancer or multiple sclerosis, like my mom. It could be worse, I guess. Sometimes I think it has to do with being alone. I'm the kind of person who likes to be alone. (He is very serious.)

Tell me what college was like for you, Mike.

I studied political science in college. I wasn't that into it, but it seemed like something that my parents, and especially my dad could approve of. I mean, they were paying for it, right? So I guess I could go into law, or politics. I've been thinking about graduate school. But I'm not sure what I want to study. Not really poli-sci. Cathy's got herself kind of set—she's studying art history in grad school. That's what she was studying when we met in Italy. But for me, I don't really know what direction to go in. It's hard for me to talk about this stuff with my mom and dad. My dad especially. I know he wants what's best for me. I know he cares. But he has these ideas about what's practical. I mean, he works for the government. And I think he chose that because it's steady and solid. I just don't think that kind of life is really for me. (Mike is pensive here.)

When you think about the future, what mood comes up? Do you see any opening? Is there anything, even if it sounds way out, that you love to do? I'm thinking of a Sufi saying translated by the poet Robert Bly: "Let the beauty we love be what we do. There are hundreds of ways to kneel and kiss the ground." What do you think about what I just said?

I like it.... Yes, actually, there is something—since I was a little kid I loved to make up stories. I had one about this boy and his dog. They talked to each other and got into all kinds of different situations. I mean, they could go anywhere—a different country, a different planet. I would illustrate these stories like a comic strip. I secretly still do. I'm always doodling and making caricatures of people. I guess you could say it's a way of kissing the ground. Maybe with my poli-sci background, I could be a political cartoonist! (Mike laughs and leans back.) I don't see any future in it, though. I wouldn't even know how to begin to get a cartoonist career off the ground.

Maybe with a little creativity you could come up with something. Are you good?

Yes... yes, I am. (He leans forward and muses. His body becomes more relaxed.)

Now, talk to me about you and your mom? What does she teach you?

Her name is Mary. We're pretty close. She's been sick a lot, though. She's very courageous. I think that's what she teaches me—courage in the face of adversity. And persistence. She never gives up. She puts her heart into everything. Like I said, she was sick a lot. She was diagnosed with multiple sclerosis when I was 10, soon after she had my sister Janie. It's been really hard for her—hard for our whole family. I always felt, as a kid, that I needed to be careful around her. You know, like not make too much noise in the house. Not bring a lot of other kids tramping through. And even now, I want her to really believe I'm OK. I don't want her to worry about me or my sister. She's so brave about everything. My mom is very passionate about life, even though she's been sick a lot. Maybe that's made her appreciate things more. She's very spiritual. Her religion is important to her. She raised me and my sister as Catholics, like I told you. (His voice is singing.)

Your dad? Who is your father for you?
Who he is for me? Secure. Strong. He doesn't show his emotions a lot. *Things* my sister and I needed when we were growing up, he really provided for us. He couldn't give us much of his time, though. And when he was there, he always seemed tired. And he worries about my mother a lot. He's someone I know I can depend on. If I were ever in a real jam, he would help me out. I think he wants me to be secure in some job... (He muses here.) One thing I really like is how much he loves my mom. With her he is pretty tender. I'd like to be closer to him. His name is Jim.

How about your sister Janie? What are you learning from her?
Learning something from my little sister? I don't think I've ever thought about her that way. Janie is more carefree than I am. She expresses her emotions more than I do. She expresses them outwardly. I wish I could be more that way. I wish I could get away with it! She doesn't worry about disappointing my parents or worrying them or anything. And the weird thing is, I don't think they really do worry about her. She's in junior high now, and I think she enjoys school more that I did. She's doing more extracurricular things. I always concentrated on grades more. Funny, she's my little sister and boys are starting to really notice her. She's cool.

What will you be looking for to know if treatment is working for you?
Well, I mean if my asthma went away that would be great. But I guess even if the attacks weren't so frequent. Or if I didn't feel so scared when they happen. That would be pretty great... What else... Well, of course if things got better with Cathy, or with my relationships with women in general, that would be amazing. Also to be able to see what I need to do next in my life. My parents feel of course like if I'm not going to grad school I should be looking for a certain kind of job. And I guess they're

right, but if I just could see what is the right thing for me.

If I asked your friend Mark to tell me about you, what would he say?
What would he tell me he counts on you for?
He'd tell you that I'm a good listener, and that I'm funny. He laughs when he's around me. He counts on me to be his friend. I'm a really count-on-able friend.

At 21, you are pretty articulate about life.
I've been thinking a lot about these things, especially since this breathing scare. It's all pretty awesome.

Mike, these next questions may seem strange to you. Part of my work with you is to show you the possibility of being a new observer, to prompt you to think some new thoughts and learn some new ways of being, so you can have some freedom to be, and freedom to act effectively in facets of life you now struggle with. This inquiry presumes that you are connected to the whole of creation, and that your healing is not a private happening. You heal for the sake of the life living through you and around you. You are a practitioner for life, practicing the art of being alive. Me too. We are partners in the dance. Now—
Who, besides yourself, will benefit from your being here? Let's say the bases in life are loaded and you are about to hit a home run—who else will come home?
(Mike sits up straight, eyes shining.) I really like that thought! It makes me realize that I'm not in this by myself, that what I do might matter to somebody else. I'll have to think about it... just like you said, some new thoughts. Thanks, Dianne! (This is the first time he calls me by name, and he is very fired up with this question.)

What is your promise for life, Mike?
You mean like a goal? or a commitment?

I mean, in your presence what will show about life, no matter what?
Who will we know ourselves to be in your presence?
I know what you're getting at, I think. What I have to offer that's special. I know there is something... something I have to give the world... but I'm not sure what exactly.

Shall I tell you what I experience in your presence?
Yes (With a shaky voice.)

In your presence, life shows as tender, awesome, and good, Mike. You show. It is so clear that to you life is a gift, and that you do not take it

for granted. With a kind of humility and openness you are searching for how to best serve and be in life. Thank you.
Thank you, Dianne.

If you want to identify me, ask me not where I live, or what I like to eat, or how I comb my hair, but ask me what I am living for, in detail, and ask me what I think is keeping me from living fully for the thing I want to live for.

Thomas Merton

Commentary on Mike as the Dance of the Elements

Each of us is the whole of the dance every moment, so every element is always present. Nothing is missing. We do not have to go someplace to find Mike. He is right here, already home. It is his birthright to be home in life. Working together, can he and I clear the way so that he can learn new ways of being big enough to be home en route? Big enough for what life is now requiring of him?

Taking a few words from each of the elements in the main text, let's look together at Mike and the Wu Shing—the five element dance. There are many associations and correlations to each element. See the text of this book, and the pages included here from our SOPHIA brochure for the range of associations. Let us begin with Water.

Water is wet, fluid. It takes the shape of whatever contains it. It flows (see p. 75). Mike, as Water, is struggling. He is in the unknown, the deep waters, the winter element—being called to listen, to be still in the midst of the inquiry. Just like bears and frogs that go deep into the dark, we too are called by the winter element to contemplation. Water is the element of reassurance that we are always in the mystery, that we are always in unknowing and that this is part of the dance. In fact, unless we are willing not to know, we will not *inquire:* we will not learn to ask and live in the powerful questions of being alive. And just as we can trust the winter to give birth to spring, we can also trust that if we stay in the unknowing it will naturally give birth to the next vision, the next seeing, the next clear distinction to act on.

In the culture that Mike, and many of us, grew up in, not a lot of time is spent in silence, in the power of the Water, in the clear flowing movement with nature. Often anxious about not knowing, we attempt to rush to early ripening—as if an apple tree in bloom could force apples to come in the spring. Mike is in the unknowing about work, about his breathing, and about his relationship to Cathy.

In treatment, the Water element will need attending, so that Mike is reassured and less afraid of what he needs to learn. The point *Greater Mountain Stream*, a source point in the Water element, will be important to incorporate, as a reminder to Mike of courage, fluidity, and the indomitable power of the force of water. The Water is the promise of easy powerful flowing. Our vitality, courage, and sexual potency are part of this dance. So is our boldness, our living of the adventure!

The **Wood** element is a tree, pure and simple. It grows up and out and down and in at the same time. Wood is about our roots and our branches. It is about the springtime, the time of new life, birth, growth, distinctions for life, a vision of possibility, a creativity rising up showing itself as the manifest kingdom. Spring is easy to see (see p.21).

Mike, as Wood, is taking seriously that he is alive and can make choices for the future—the future of his work life, his love life, his wellbeing, his gift to what is yet to be. He is growing, and just by virtue of his coming for treatment he is taking action to get some direction and clearer perception, some ease and balance. He is learning to see himself as unique and distinct from his family, especially regarding a life's work as distinct from his father's. It may be that seeing on every level will open up—hindsight, foresight, insight, nearsight. He cannot yet quite imagine really living his creativity and making a livelihood.

In Mike's presence I am reminded of certain points in the Wood element—for example, *Wilderness Mound*, to remind Mike that he can already see and that he has the capability of wise judgment; *Crooked Spring*, to remind him how trustworthy, like nature, he is.

After the winter of not knowing comes the spring of aliveness and spontaneous direction. In the presence of the squawk—the symptom called asthma—rather than anger and fear as a reaction, Mike could learn to embrace the shout from his body as a call to life. The symptom can then readily disappear once there is no resistance holding it in place. New openings like the springtime flowers start to show, a kind of hope and beauty of new beginnings. And we, as beginners, learn to discern how to dance the spring into life. Mike is like the tree, simple and mighty at once.

Fire is warmth and light. The sun is the source of Fire (p.35). Mike, as the Fire element, has a strength and a struggle. The strength is clear. He is fundamentally joyful: he deeply knows life to be a dance, a dance of partnership. In his presence there is enthusiasm, laughter, a certain lightness of being, even though he has serious concerns. He is joyful and serious all at once. The expression of love for life is heartfelt. He is hearty in his warmth. Mike's struggle shows in his pain over intimacy and sex with Cathy. Sex is a basic human concern. It could be said that sex is a deep kind of touch, a sharing of one's senses, one's condition for being, one's embodiment. Touch is the sense most associated with Fire.

Mike's distress exemplifies the distress of the culture. Sex in many instances has become a frivolous conversation fraught with ambiguities and oppositions, sinful versus sacred, sport versus solemn ritual, game versus lifelong commitment, abuse versus gift. Mike, at 21, lives in a culture of remnants; he must construct his own embodied discourse about intimacy and lovemaking amidst a cacophony of diverse, often opposing thoughts. He is beginning to recognize that it is his voice and listening heart that create the conversations meaningful to him and life around him. He can and does and must construct meanings for being alive. He gets to speak into the prevailing cultural wind what he holds passionately, what he deems most dear.

Mike is learning with Cathy, and she with him. They are partners, at least for now. Whether they stay together as married mates or not doesn't matter. What matters is that as fellow travelers they love one another, seeking to be helpmates—whatever the form from here—for the unique expression that lives through each of them. Even if they never see each other again, what will remain so is that they have helped each other along the way. Fire is the promise of friendship, the camaraderie of existence. I have no doubt that treating Mike in Fire will serve him powerfully well. The relationship of Fire to Water is crucial, since water only flows easily when it is warm enough; otherwise it is ice.

Earth is the ground beneath our feet (see p.51). Mike, as the Earth element, is full and fertile. The Scriptural passage, "by their fruits you will know them," comes to mind in his presence. He cares about what happens with people and is thoughtful about them. His concerns have a kind of tenderness and consideration, a sweet caring about the life around him. For example, the way he responds about his mom, his sister, his grandmother show a certain simpatico. Nourishment is a facet of Earth, both being nourished and being nourishing. Mike has this well established. It is clear in his presence.

The Earth, according to the classic texts, is also the creator of connections and the holder of all transition. It is the mother, the center, an equilibrium/middle, official residence for all of the changes called life. Mike is right in the midst of a transition—no longer in college, not yet in work; no longer in a committed relationship with Cathy, yet not quite out of it, either; no longer a boy about his physical well-being, yet not quite a man about his mortality. During our initial interview, whenever he made a connection his whole body relaxed. For example, when he recognized that he was still living his historical narrative about sex being bad, something to get over with quickly, he physically breathed easier. It was as though a new physical comfort is now possible. When he connected breathing with the rest of his life, a new thoughtfulness became possible.

Certain points on the Earth pathways are clear in Mike's presence, like Mike's offerings to life; *Great Enveloping, Encircling Glory, Basket Gate, Abundant Splendor, People Welcome.* Since food is a gift from the Earth, it is good to see that Mike relishes it and likes to prepare it for others. He is compassionate, tenderly thoughtful, and considerate of those in life with him. When he realized that his healing would matter to all of us, that his home run would bring us home, he gladdened.

Metal (see p.63) is the elemental salt of the earth, the crystalline clarity of the jewel, the long-lasting richness of life, the endurance of beauty. Mike, as Metal, knows life, like the air we breathe, to be a precious gift. This labeled illness, asthma, serves to remind him even at such a young age of the wonder of being alive, of the wonder of being able to do easily the simple things like breathing. Breath is a matter of life and death for all of us. Without breath for four minutes, we would not be here. It is profoundly associated with the Ch'i, the Life Force itself—that without which we are dead. Our vital impulse, the rhythmic order of inhale, exhale, inspire, out-spire, the alternating pulse of the heavenly Ch'i is held by the awesome power to breathe. The Metal element is about amazement, astonishment, appreciation.

Metal is thus the connection with the father, with the heavens, in the way that Earth is the connection with the mother. Mike received from his grandmother, his father's mother, a confidence and sense of himself, a sense of value and worth. This woman had also raised his father, yet somehow Mike had missed him. Some of Mike's cry is for his father. Part of my work with Mike in the treatment room will be to draw a distinction between the phenomenon father and the conclusion father, so that Mike can see his father newly. Then he can acknowledge him for the wonder he is, just as he is—the same acknowledgment as when Mike spoke of the Muir Woods as taking his breath away. He said it in awe and wonder; it was a bow to life, a bow to the phenomenon with no conclusion but awe. Mike had this same reverence in speaking of the sunrise and sunset, the same respect when speaking of his grandmother.

Mike is so clear about the gifts and beauty of existence. One of Mike's main questions about life is how will he serve, what is the best expression, the best use of him. What is the beauty he loves, so that can be what he does for his life's work? What is his gift to offer? And, doesn't the squawk called asthma, i.e., difficulty in breathing, call him to take seriously what he will breathe into life.

Each of us is a bowing servant between heaven and earth, being called with dignity and honor to our unique bow, bearing for each other whatever is ours to bear, offering to each other what we have to give. Mike, through the intensity of the symptom asthma, is having to take seriously the unique breath of life that is his to inspire, for all of our sakes.

> *gateway of being: open your being, awaken,*
> *learn then to be, begin to carve your face,*
> *develop your elements, and keep your vision*
> *keen to look at my face, as I at yours,*
> *keen to look full at life right through to death,*
> *faces of sea, of bread, of rock, of fountain,*
> *the spring of origin which will dissolve our faces*
> *in the nameless face, existence without face*
> *the inexpressible presence of presences....*
> **Octavio Paz**
> ***The Sunstone***

Treatments

For the ***first treatment***, I used points on Mike's back, known as Associated Effect Points, in the Water element pathway of the bladder. This is the mighty Amazon River of pathways, being the most extensive meridian with 67 points: wonderful points corresponding to all the elements. (For this reason, they are also sometimes known as the Correspondence Points.) I think of this treatment as being like a break-shot in pool, where the balls are all clumped together and the first action is to open them up on the table, pocket a few, and set others up for pocketing. It is quite a good image for Mike's first needles. Another image is that of spring winds which clear out all the old debris; they make way for the new life of the arriving springtime. Treating these points clears the way so that Mike's birth-right, the nature of the distinct unique expression of Life that he is, can come forth with strength and clarity.

Points used:
III 13(metal), 14(fire), 15(fire), 18(wood), 20(earth), 23(water).
Three moxa on Governor Vessel 4, *Gate of Life* to support what I did with the needles.

After the first treatment, Mike saw Cathy. It was an unexpected visit. She had surprised him and come home for the weekend. He told her about our session together, and they talked in a deeper way than they ever had. They were intimate in a new and easier way, realizing that it might take time to learn to really make love with each other. She told him that she had changed her mind about being with other guys, and she wanted to be steady with him. Mike was overjoyed! I asked if he noticed anything else since the first treatment. He told me he was particularly tired the first day and a half, then just felt good the whole rest of the time. His breathing was about the same, though he said he was not as concerned about it as he had been.

The **second treatment** included a recheck of the akabanes to see if the six pathways that were initially out of balance still were. Numbers IV (kidneys) and III (bladder), both Water element meridians, came into balance after the "break-shot." The others, however, were still off: I (heart) to the right, V (heart protector-circulation sex) to the right, VI (three heater) to the left, all three of those in the Fire element. IX (lungs) in the Metal element remained off to the left. In order to have ease since each of these main pathways is bilateral, they need to be in balance bilaterally. Many squawks can arise when one or more pathways are calling for balancing.

I 5 — joining point — *Penetrating Inside*
V 6 — joining point — *Inner Frontier Gate*
VI 5 — joining point — *Outer Frontier Gate*
IX 7 — joining point — *Narrow Defile*

Also part of the second treatment was to massage the center pulse back into the center. It had been slightly off to the south. This centering is very important for Mike's focus and balance. It was also important to note that the Water element responded immediately; we can simply observe how the Water pulses hold without having to touch them directly for now.

Third treatment testing showed that the akabanes held very well, and Mike's pulses were exhibiting a robust, easier flowing quality all around the cycle—like a strong sigh of relief and ease throughout. His Fire pulses were particularly steady and vigorous. The pulse of the lungs, the official (in Metal) of the great receiving of the pure Ch'i from the heavens, was also stronger. This was good news since the breath and breathing are deeply attended by the Ch'i associated with this pathway, and one of Mike's profound concerns is his breathing. Since the second treatment he had noticed that he was craving spicy food more than usual. Spice is the taste associated with Metal.

The third treatment was a simple entry-exit point combination in Fire on the circulation sex-heart protector pathway. The points used were V 1, *Heavenly Pond*, which also is thought of as a window in that Fire meridian, an opening, a freeing up; and V 9, *Rushing into the Middle*, a kind of indomitable presence of life as we plunge headlong into the day. It is also the Wood point of that Fire pathway. It takes a good strong Wood to make a good strong Fire. So many of Mike's concerns, both sexually and in terms of his life's work, are addressed by needling these points, points that he has had his whole life long. By putting a needle in, all I am doing is reminding him of who he already is as a heavenly pond, an opening, a window, an entrance for life. Who he already is as rushing into the middle, a surge of indomitable life force presenting himself for the whole of the dance.

After the third treatment, Mike observed that he felt "lighter." He had the same concerns, and yet he was easier, more relaxed. He said he kept sighing a lot. He had had some talks with his father about the future, and had found himself reassuring his father! To his astonishment, he discovered that his father was also thinking about the future, and a career change. Mike's mother and sister were both urging him on to do what he really wanted to do in the cartoon world, even if it meant waiting tables for a while to earn his keep. Mike also observed that he is using less asthma medicine, even going for two days without using the inhaler. He is increasingly enthusiastic, and according to his sister, more fun.

When healing begins to show in the familiar world around us, we know that we are arriving; when life around us shows up with renewed vitality, spontaneity and joy! We heal for the sake of each other. This simplicity is staggering. Cathy comments about how much more available Mike is, even over the telephone, and how much happier she is in his presence now.

The fourth treatment was also in the Fire element—in the three heater (VI). VI 1 *Rushing the Frontier Gate*, VI 22 *Harmony Bone*, VI 23 *Silk Bamboo Hollow*. These points in this official of Fire call to the power of the three heater to provide the milieu for wholeness, to create the heat and light necessary for living. Without illumination we cannot see, without warmth we cannot touch, without joy we cannot trust. Fire is a life principle, a compelling, passionate, radiant brilliance. It serves Mike well to support the Fire, to call on its strength and bring it into balance. The spirit of these points takes in both beauty and purposefulness. Silk and bamboo are both wondrous gifts of nature, beautiful and wonderfully useful—like Mike. Bone is a translation of what is essential, the bones of life, and harmony brings concord, beauty, melody to life, life in concert. *Rushing the Frontier Gate*, as the entrance point, calls past the edge of Mike's personal limiting conclusions into an indomitable movement of promise and possibility.

As Mike and I continue to work together, he is becoming a keen observer of life, both as it lives through him and as it lives through all those around him. As he learns new steps in the dance of life, and as he dances them more powerfully and gracefully, Mike comes to know himself as practitioner, making openings and creating possibilities for others. In essence, the work Mike and I do together is a calling to remember. I, as practitioner for life, call him to remember who he is — already healed, already whole, already home. By remembering, he as practitioner for life, calls us all home.

Chapter Ten

Vignettes

Vignettes

Each of these vignettes is meant to be read as a parable: a story of others, which in the reading becomes a learning, a treatment for the reader. Each shows some new possibility of being alive.

Rose is 89 years old and recently had eye surgery that left her unable to see. She is, to me, a striking reminder of the possibility that aging and "saging" go together. Her sageliness is readily apparent: when I asked her was she eager to get back her sight, she hesitated and said that she wasn't so sure. I, a bit astonished, listened while she told me what she was learning without the eye-vision she had taken for granted. She ended by saying that of course she wanted seeing eyes again, yet also to always remember the "arrogance of the sighted." For Rose, who comes for treatment at the change of seasons, acupuncture helps her hold steady through all the uncharted changes of her aging. She has no map, nor do I. She has only the territory of each day in creation as she lives it. We are pals and partners. Treating her, I am reminded that the care and touching she gets from me is crucial for her continuing knowing of herself in her embodied existence. I often use points in the Wood element to support Rose—*Valiant Stream* to remind her of her courageous on-going aliveness; *Great Esteem* to call her to the gift she brings to all of us through the dignity of her life. One of Rose's offerings to me, and therefore to you as I tell you, is in the form of a little paperback book written by Florida Scott-Maxwell. The book is called *The Measure of My Days*, written when the author was 82 years old.

When a new disability arrives I look about to see if death has come, and I call quietly, "Death, is that you? Are you there?" So far the disability has answered, "Don't be silly, it's me."

> **Florida Scott-Maxwell**
> ***The Measure of My Days***

Diana is 48 years old, an executive in a business corporation. When we first met, half-way through the initial exam, she blurted out, "You seem so joyful. How do you do that?" I asked her if she was asking out of curiosity—if so then I would not respond to the question. If she was asking so that the answer would really serve her, then I would answer. I thought that since she did not come for me to "pussy-foot" with her, I would talk straight, and from the beginning of our connection would offer what I think are powerful distinctions for being alive. She was a little shocked at first, never having heard these distinctions. Then she said, very graciously, that she would listen in the same way a player listens to a coach. I was grateful and proceeded to tell her that I am "in training" to make sure that wherever I am the dance of the five elements will show, and that one of the elements is Fire, associated with light, warmth, heart, partnership, joy. I figure we need more joy on this creaky old earth, so I practice joy. Diana lit up as she listened. She had come to me because she had heard that acupuncture treatment could help with "stress." She realized that what she was calling "stressful" was a conclusion about certain phenomena in her work life. The phenomena were simple things: for instance, when she would arrive at work in the morning, no one smiled or looked up to greet her. The mood of her fellow workers was solemn and serious with very little joy. Diana had forgotten that she has something to offer to change that—forgotten that when she brings joy present an ease and camaraderie become available for everyone, including Diana! The points *Relax and Joy, Utmost Source, Rushing into the Middle,* and *Outer Frontier Gate* (in the Fire element) are wonderful points to help Diana embody a lightness of being. They enhance her ongoing learning of life as a dance in which she is integral as dancer.

If you haven't been fed, be bread.
Sufi saying

Jason is 12 years old. He started treatment when he was 8, after his mother observed him having a "hard time" in school. He agreed. What that meant for Jason, in his own words, was that "being in school is like riding on a bumper car. Every moment I might get hit by someone or run into someone... not like really hit, more like shaken up. Then I get really mad and cause trouble." He was waking up every morning with pains in his belly and feeling "sick"—sick like car-sick, queasy and unsettled. In being with Jason I soon discovered his love and passion for music. He fancied himself as a rock star (and he had not told anyone but his friend Randy). I asked for a demonstration and he gave me one of a song he had written! "Do you get to sing in school?" "No." "Could you?" "Maybe." I then asked him if he thought it was possible to "sing" his studies. He knew what I meant! "Like inside my head?" "Yes, like that." The element most calling for balancing for Jason is Earth. The Earth's gifts are many, especially for Jason. Earth brings a deep knowing that "I am connected and I belong" to the whole. Its sound is singing, the sweet rhythmic song of life as One. Its focus is the thoughtful, compassionate, nourishing. For Jason, I include points like *Abundant Splendor, Great Oneness, Not at Ease, Inner Courtyard, Heavenly Pivot, People Welcome,* and *Great Enveloping.* These are all on the Earth pathways. (Jason is fine with the needles. Some children are not, in which case I use only moxa or finger pressure on the point.) He reports being less "bumpy"; he doesn't awaken with a "belly ache" anymore and he has formed a little rock group called "The Points"! He "might" let me sing with them some day!

> *I celebrate myself, and sing myself,*
> *And what I assume, you shall assume,*
> *For every atom belonging to me as good as belongs to you.*
> **Walt Whitman**
> ***Song of Myself***

Linda is 28 years old, an editor of an arts magazine. She had "tried" acupuncture a few years ago with a practitioner who moved to another town. Linda's first statement was, "I am so lonely, I don't know what to do. Everyone I try to connect with ends up disliking me." I could hear immediately that the conversation she was constructing of her life, a conversation of disconnection, was too small to live in; she could not "get home from there." The conversation was too constricting for her *and* others around her, especially those she was "trying" to connect with. Words *are* needles, I say. Words are treatments. I also take very seriously the theme from Heidegger, the philosopher, that our forgetfulness of being is in our speaking. Given that Linda is an editor, she knows the potency of words. Yet she wasn't hearing her own narrative, nor was she observing that her suffering was connected with it. For example, the word "try" lives in a conversation of failure, of "can't," of "difficult." For Linda there is freedom in declaring herself a beginner in the arena of partnership. For her to say that she is "not practiced" gives her more room to design a new practice of partnering. There is more freedom here than in her other conversation of "trying," or saying that something is hard. The Water element is associated with the unknowing, with the mysteries of being alive, and with the fortuitous nature of life. Fear and courage are part of it, and a willingness to listen deeply to what is essential. This is the winter element that calls us deep into the dark—also a part of life. It calls us to keep listening for possibility every moment. Points like *Greater Mountain Stream, Illumi-*

nated Sea, Through the Valley—all in the Water element—are wonderful to incorporate into Linda's treatment. Now Linda is more peaceful in herself more of the time. She is learning to let herself be a beginner, and to say it. She is also recognizing that her perception that others dislike her may simply be an unedited story that she is telling.

> **O to be self-balanced for contingencies,**
> **To confront night, storms, hunger, ridicule,**
> **accidents, rebuffs, as the trees and animals do.**
> **Walt Whitman**

I treat Harry, and have for almost eight years now. When the news came that one of his children, Joseph, had fallen to his death in a climbing accident, Harry called me. It was 2:30 in the morning. To me, the one unbearable happening had occurred—a child had died while the parents were alive. What is there to speak in this unendurable circumstance? I am Harry's friend, his practitioner. What is my practice in this moment? It must be to practice a bow to the awesomeness of this dance of existence, to speak compassionate sorrow, not sentimentality for what is asked of us beings of the human sort. "A condition of complete simplicity (Costing not less than everything)" writes T.S.Eliot. Harry is face to face with the mortality that belongs to all of us through his son, Joseph. When Eric Clapton's young son fell out a window to his death, his father turned the excruciating suffering into an offering in the form of a song, *Tears In Heaven*. The most I can say is thank you to Harry for allowing me to tend him in this heartbreaking moment, for permitting me the privilege of being with him in his grief. "Dona nobis pacem — Grant us peace." I have used the points *Utmost Source, Spirit Gate,* and *Spirit Path,* all on the Heart pathway, to help Harry with his pain. Also, the *Joining of the Valleys* on the pathway of the great letting go, the large intestine.

> **...then I turn the pain of absence into an offering to God.**
> **Sometimes that's all I have to offer...**
> **Brother Patrick**
> **in *Blue Highways***
> **by William Least Heat Moon**

Gwen is 6 years old. At the time of this writing I have seen her through a whole cycle of seasons. She came originally because of "awful, almost-every-day headaches," particularly over her right eye. She would get sick and throw up. Western medicine offered temporary relief with medication, yet nothing changed the frequency or intensity. All medical tests, including of her vision, were fine. Gwen's mother and father were very concerned, quite beside themselves. Both of them are busy judges, and though they continually make discernments in the judicial world, they couldn't see what to do for their girl. Gwen first said, "My mommy is mad at me. She is mad because my head hurts. I am mad too." The gift of the Wood element is the gift of vision, of opening toward the future, of creativity and direction, of clear perception, of the springtime. Gwen's symptom, the headache, the "squawk," was not a problem that needed "fixing." It was a call from her young Bodymindspirit, a call to see the power and possibility of the rising-up Ch'i of the springtime element, a call to bring ease, balance and peace. The shout of the symptom was showing up not only via Gwen's head, but also in the frustration and anger around her about what to do. In this medicine I practice, that is to say this way at looking at life, a struggling to see is the same as the emotion "anger." We are angry only when we cannot see, only when we do not have a vision of possibility. With Gwen I use points to clear the Wood element, for example *Flowing Valley, Eye Window, Sun and Moon, Bright and Clear, Wilderness Mound, Happy Calm*, and *Crooked Spring*. Gwen comes at the change of seasons now. I do a little moxa, sometimes a needle. She rarely has a headache anymore. She writes poetry and smiles a lot. The whole family is easier. It's a home-run! The bases are loaded, and we all come home!

> **alive we're alive)**
> **we're wonderful one times one**
> **e.e. cummings**
> **"if everything happens that**
> **can't be done"**

Margaret is a woman, 31 years old. She is a homemaker, and she loves her two children and husband "madly"—"I'm bats over them." She found out that her husband was having an affair with a woman at work. When Margaret first came for treatment, she said things like "I'm no good," "I have no self esteem," "I don't care if I live or die," "Nothing matters any more," "I can hardly focus on my children," "I am desperate." All the apparent certainties of life had been shattered: she was face-front with daily living, unable to observe anything but brokenness. Physically she felt that she had "no energy," just a pervading fatigue and disinterest. As she cried and railed at the circumstances, unable to see how to go from here, I could hear her submerged shout of frustration. The points *Foot above Tears* and *Head above Tears* in the Wood element are powerful reminders for Margaret that she is alive, while in the midst of big life changes that she did not bargain for.

The point *Hard Bargain* in Earth is good grounding for her so she can hold steady with the children. Also the point *Great Esteem,* in Wood, serves to call her to her dignity and clarity so that she can, together with her husband, work out something beyond the pain and brokenness. *Sun and Moon,* also in Wood, reminds her of a bigger vision and possibilities not easily seen in a "local" view. She now knows that when she can be an observer and not get caught up in the drama of her own reactions, she is more effective. She can see that, for the sake of the children, she must be creative, must not let herself fall into despair and resignation with no hope for the future. *Gate of Hope and Happy Calm*—also in the element of Wood, the element of springtime—strengthen Margaret to remember who she is even though she does not like the circumstances.

> **My barn having burned to the ground**
> **I can now see the moon.**
> **Old Chinese Sage**

Alan is a 70 year old gentleman whose wife, Anne, died a year ago. He was holding her hand when she breathed her last breath. It was excruciating for him to let her go. They had been sweethearts for 50 years, knowing that the day would come that one of them would not be here when the other was. When he first came to me for treatment, he was "very blue." Alan was referred for acupuncture by his therapist, who thought he was suicidal. I could see that he was stricken, both grief stricken and lost without his mate. He reminded me of geese, of how when one has fallen, the other never mates again. This gentleman embodies the wondrous phenomenon of mourning, the awesomeness of sorrow.

I use points in the great Metal element to help Alan dance in his valley of tears; points in the pathway of the great letting go (the large intestine); and points in the pathway of the great receiving of the pure Ch'i from the heavens (the lungs). The point called *Joining of the Valleys* helps him tremendously. After I did that point, he recalled that in the Catholic tradition of his youth, there were three sets of mysteries, not only the Sorrowful, but also the Joyful and the Glorious. This comforted him. Another powerful point for Alan is called *Wail of Grief,* reminding us that lamentation is elemental: we all will weep and lament at some moment along the way. In the midst of his sorrow, Alan had a dream of sitting by Anne's bed, holding her hand and berating himself for not having been a more thoughtful, loving, compassionate husband. Suddenly he heard the words, "You are all on a journey home. The one thing of importance is that during this time you all help one another. You are each other's keepers." He said it seemed that his entire body was taken over by a Presence (his capital P) far greater than his own with a compassion and love beyond words. He calls his life a "joint venture with God."

Daniel is a 17-year-old young man, African-American, who at the age of 14 was in a horrible car accident in which his father was killed and Daniel was left in a coma. He wasn't expected to recover. He rallied and did regain a lot of his physical strength, though his right arm and leg are partially paralyzed. While in the coma, Daniel heard conversations that he still remembers. He pleaded with me to let other people know that what is said in a sickroom, even if it seems that the person can't hear or isn't responding, *is* important. For instance his mom would croon to him, the old spirituals they always sang in his family's church. She'd speak to him as though he were hearing her. Others would come in and talk about him as though he were not there. Daniel is sure that his mom saved his life by calling to him to come back to her, saying that she was so sad his dad was gone, she couldn't bear it if he were to leave too. He told me that he returned for her sake. Daniel is such a loving presence. He genuinely does live for the sake of others, always looking to see how he can be of assistance. Treatment is an ongoing support. I often go to points on the Governor Vessel — the great call to life, and the Conception Vessel — the great response to the call to life, especially *Gate of Life* on the Governor Vessel and *First Gate* or *Stone Gate* on the Conception Vessel. There are lots of gates in different places on the body, passageways, gateways. Needling a gate reminds Daniel of who he is as a portal for life.

I'm here by the gate.
Maybe you'll throw open a door and call....
By this gate Kings are waiting with me.
Rumi

Rick is 28 years old, a musician who is gay and two years ago found out that he is "positive" for HIV, the virus that causes AIDS. He had discovered some purplish spots on his thigh. The diagnosis was Kaposi's sarcoma. Many of his friends in the gay community who are also HIV-positive told him that acupuncture was a big help to them—a help to heal, to ease the fear, to keep a balance, and to be stronger. When Rick first arrived for treatment, he had just read *And the Band Played On,* the Randy Shilts book in which a young man spoke about the virus as being like a lover, calling him to life's precious moments and reminding him that life is for loving. Rick was entertaining seriously the possibility that the virus was a gift and that his task was to live wisely, with respect for the virus as though it were a guest in the house. For Rick's mother and father, the fact of their son's homosexuality was deeply shocking, and even more terrifying for them was their concern that he might get AIDS. He hadn't told them of the blood test result.

For Rick, acupuncture treatment is a haven, a respite from what he perceives as a pervading conversation of illness in his community. I work with him in the Water element using points like *Rich for the Vitals, Diaphragm Gate of Vitality, Receive and Support, Prosperous Gate, Penetrating the Valley, Supporting Mountain,* and *Equilibrium Middle.* I coach him to keep unhooking any conclusions he has drawn about himself, about the labels "AIDS" and "HIV." I have seen labels "become" *the* conversation about who the person is and yet, it is never the symptom that has the person. It is the person who has the symptom. Labels and conclusions often get in the way of fully living and experiencing our bodies this moment. A medical test, no matter how high tech, cannot determine our experience of being alive unless we say so.

One sure concern that comes up in the AIDS conversation is the recognition that we are mortals, who only dwell here on the earth for a while, in the form we know ourselves to be. Rick has begun to talk with his folks about their fears for him and themselves. They are closer than they have ever been, holding back nothing. They cherish each other, expressing their love.

> *At his death, Joe's dad told his son, "Never be embarrassed about your love, ever, son. Make sure you tell your friends too. Love is what life is for."*
> **Joe, in the treatment room**
> **talking about his dad, 1990**

MANY OTHERS COME FOR TREATMENT:

Jed, a 55-year-old gentleman who suffers from "back trouble" and sleep difficulties, and whose work "is" his life; Jean, a 38-year-old physician of African-American and Spanish ancestry who is "caught" in a cultural conversation uncertain where she wants to live and work; Gay, 44-year-old woman artist who feels "stuck," unable to face a canvas without panicking and thinking of herself as a failure. She also forces herself to throw up after eating in order to stay "model thin"; Bill, 46-year-old business man who travels weekly in "high stress" conditions and "cannot" slow down or relax without alcohol which then gives him a headache; Madeline, age 50, who on turning 50 gained 12 pounds in a month, lost her high-paying military job, and is in a "crisis" about her future; Jeanne, age 31, with "Crohn's disease." High amounts of cortisone cause her body to retain fluid and her face to be "moon-like"; JJ, a 3-year-old boy who periodically gets a fever, rapid breathing, serious wheezing and coughing; Pam, age 33, who wants to get pregnant and has been trying for two years; Jack, age 54, who had cosmetic surgery on his eyes and "has not been right since"; Phil, age 38, who got addicted to cocaine and lost custody of his children over it, in great pain over his broken family; Marianne, 53 years old, diagnosed as having multiple sclerosis, who comes in from Bermuda for treatment at regular monthly intervals; Mary, age 60, wanting support for strength and balance after successful chemotherapy for breast cancer; Matthew, Mary's husband, 63 years old, just retired and still in some shock over Mary's illness. Both want help with their sex life which had been wonderful until the cancer treatment "took the stuffing out of them"; Jake, age 6, who was in a devastating car accident that left him unable to see, to speak, to walk. His mother died in the crash.

I love this life. I am moved by the privilege of being with others, bearing witness to their sufferings and offerings, "in-seeing" the courage that it takes to keep being alive until we are dead. My promise is that no matter what, wherever I am, life will show as a possibility for others. Acupuncture helps me to keep my promise. It is ongoing training. Keeping my promise is a daily practice. I am a practitioner for life, practicing the art of being alive. So are you.

Appendix

Appendix 1

Who is Dianne M. Connelly?

For me, Acupuncture is a continual challenge to grow and understand humanity. A person comes to me asking for help and oftentimes in desperation. I stretch to know who that person is and what she needs for her life to be healthy and fruitful. I question whether I can really come to know her needs clearly. I question whether I can understand my own needs clearly. My own life goes through ups and downs, a roller coaster of the human condition. How can I be of service to someone? Am I thinking I am Lady Bountiful with answers to give? Do I allow my own life force to flow strong and pure? What do I do with my own needs and my own troubles when I am with a patient? Am I a healer?

All these questions, and more, confront me in my profession. I am Dianne—the culmination of the 30 years experience I've lived. I am Dianne before I am the Acupuncturist. I am insecurity and confidence, winces and grins, beast and beauty. Some things that are important to me are keeping life's games out front where I can see them and call them, making sure that hidden expectations get *found out*, struggling to be clear and pure in my love. I am vulnerable; I want to be loved; I get mighty angry. I sometimes feel sorry for myself, worthless, proud.

As an Acupuncturist I forget my personal history. A person comes in for an examination and I feel drawn into her life story. I listen carefully. No one else in the world exists. Like Penelope, she weaves, and I watch to see what she is weaving—looking for the colors, the designs, the textures. I ask her who she is, absorbed in her. I write what she tells me and what I see. Sometimes her story is horrifying and I feel dismay; still, I record it as she says. Sometimes the story is sad and full of longing; still, it belongs to her, and I learn to let it be hers without having to make it mine too. Sometimes the story is obscure and complex, sometimes knotted and strange, yet there are no judgements and no blame to be given. I am often aware of the intimacy in an examination, a closeness, feeling things the way another feels them.

There are times when it is difficult for me to stay clear. Once in an examination with someone who was very hostile, I began to take it personally rather than see the hostility as a symptom and a cry for help. Because I am in a group practice, I call on my colleagues to help understand what is happening. With another person who complained and whined through the entire two and one half hour examination, I felt drained and picked up her symptom of nausea. This is an interesting phenomenon . . . the picking up of a patient's symptoms: It seems to happen most frequently with student Acupuncturists who are just beginning to take on responsibility in the treatment room. Perhaps it is the anxiety and the tension within, perhaps it is a clash of imbalance between patient and practitioner, perhaps it is a low defense mechanism; whatever it is, the symptom is very real.

I remember one night, in my early days of Acupuncture, treating a woman who had a persistent pain in the area of her left ovary. That evening for about an hour and a half, I had a pain of the same description over my left ovary. That was the first and only time that I have ever had a pain there like that. I think that, because the exam and treatment work on such a basic deep level of energy, and because there is an intense interchange between patient and practitioner, if the practitioner is not in top form, she is apt to take the patient's symptoms onto herself. This is one reason why it is so necessary for a practitioner to stay clear and balanced. It is not so strange, though, that symptoms get exchanged, even though they are not contagious in a traditional sense. In other life situations like love relationships, one moody, upset partner can quickly become two, if the other partner is not able to stay clear or starts to take the upset upon herself.

Now, in the midst of all this, you might ask . . . if you're just a normal person with ups and downs and imperfections, how can you be an objective Acupuncturist? How do you know that the information you find from the patient is not your own projection? Good question. I think there is no such thing as an objective anything, including an objective Acupuncturist. There is always something of me in what I do. Just as the patient is a unique individual, recapitulating her life every moment, I, too, am a unique individual, recapitulating my life every moment. With these questions I am reminded of Margaret Mead, whose anthropological field work is not that of an uninvolved observer . . . the people she studies experience her as a person warm and loving. In anthropological circles she is often taken to task for her *unscientific* approach, yet she has taught us at least as much as if not more than any anthropologist about peoples and humanity. I would be presumptuous to think of myself as a Margaret Mead of Acupuncture, but I do emulate the spirit with which she works.

The only thing that I can be sure of in myself is whether I am being true at every moment. If I am, then I am being honest whatever I am doing. For me to be objective is to be clear. If I need to know whether or not I am projecting on a patient, I ask her about it. It is nearly always possible to check out any doubt by asking. If I am loving, open and warm ... trying to stay as clear as I can, that is all that I can do to insure the validity of my perceptions and abilities as an Acupuncture practitioner.

It makes so much innate sense to me that the body should follow a process predicated on Nature and her cycles. It feels right that harmony and balance be used as the language of health; and that human beings basically want to be healthy in bodymindspirit, seeking balance and harmony. I trust my bodymindspirit. Sometimes I fail.

In the treatment room with a person, I feel an awesome responsibility. I think it has to do with awareness of the power in the Life Force. Each treatment is a cosmic task and requires my utmost concentration. I love the intensity and the integrity demanded of me by my profession. It is more than a job. It is a highly articulated focus on the unity of life. It requires me to be both artist and scientist, continually synthesizing the composite of human experience. It is a life's dream.

Does Acupuncture work or aren't you just biased because you have a personal stake in it? Can it be proven?

Some hours and days I am an agnostic, thinking *Energy—if there is an Energy, let me feel you in the pulses—if there are such things as pulses!!* Yet, in spite of my occasional skeptical self, something happens that creates more health. This is true even if the patient is skeptical too—a pain disappears, a symptom changes, a feeling of well-being takes over. It seems to be neither hypnosis, nor placebo, nor belief that moves the Energy through blockage. For thousands of years the Chinese have been doing Acupuncture asking not so much the Western scientific *why* it works, but the Eastern query of *how* it works and what the skills are to that *how!* Perhaps one day science will answer its demand for proof of this healing system, much as it learned to answer the questions about blood flow in the days when the idea of a circulatory system was anathema to a scientific mind.

Personally I won't mind if or when science finds proof that Acupuncture is as real as the Chinese have for centuries known it to be, yet it would be a welcome affirmation.

Appendix 2

Postscript

I am an Acupuncture practitioner . . . but this was not always true. My own process of growth in the learning of this ancient art has been profound. It is one thing to say that since childhood I have wanted to be a healer and quite another thing to actually store up enough personal power to be a healer. I have had to learn to see—to really see, and it is as though I have been blind my whole life until now. I have had to learn to hear—to listen and perceive with exquisite acuity the sounds of health and illness, the words of life and death. I have had to learn to ask the things that are of the essence of living— the basic simple profound questions that give the information of what a person has created for herself in daily life. I have had to learn to feel—not just the textures and temperatures but the Life Force of a person, to feel the most intimate basic thrust within—the life energy. When I say *I have had* I do not mean it past tense. I mean that I have now a start and that I am only just beginning to learn what it is to be a person who cares for life—a healer.

Postscript 1990

This book you are reading, *Traditional Acupuncture: The Law of the Five Elements*, was written in 1975 as a Ph.D. project for The Union Graduate School—The Union for Experimenting Colleges and Universities. Little did I know then that sixteen years later thousands of people would be reading this book and finding its themes and information useful. It continues to provide an introduction to the healing work we do at the Traditional Acupuncture Institute in Columbia, Maryland.

Recently I wrote a second book, *All Sickness Is Home Sickness.* It too, is about healing. In the introduction I explain its purpose: "Inherent in the context of traditional acupuncture, in the body of information and interpretation, . . . is a context for being alive, for healing. . . . as in my first book, I intend to make available that vision—that is, the visionary design and the possibility for life that is inherent in acupuncture—not just for acupuncturists, students, patients, and health care practitioners, but for everyone engaged in being alive."

My life is about serving my patients, sharing my work with students of acupuncture, and being part of the Institute's new SOPHIA program (School of Philosophy and Healing in Action), which applies this vision in the everyday world. In SOPHIA, laypersons participate in a powerful discourse based on the ancient Chinese distinctions for life, learning concepts and skills through which they can respond to the challenges of the new millenium. Students in the Institute's acupuncture training program also learn to embody SOPHIA's themes: "to come to life more fully so as to serve life more wisely and more nobly," and "all work is world work."

So since 1975 I have continued to practice, to write (including a regular editor's note in *The Journal of Traditional Acupuncture*), to teach, and to present workshops and lectures on SOPHIA themes. And, Dear Readers, with you, I continue in this great dance of Life. Together we are bowing servants, caring for Life, and ever opening to the myriad possibilities of being alive.

—Dianne M. Connelly

THE MERIDIANS OF CH'I ENERGY

ILLUSTRATING THE ACUPUNCTURE POINTS OF THE FOURTEEN MAJOR MERIDIANS

PROFESSOR J.R. WORSLEY MASTER & DOCTOR OF ACUPUNCTURE M. Ac., DR. Ac., F.C.C. Ac. (CHINA), F. R. Ac. PRESIDENT: COLLEGE CHINESE ACUPUNCTURE (U.K.)

ANTERIOR TORSO

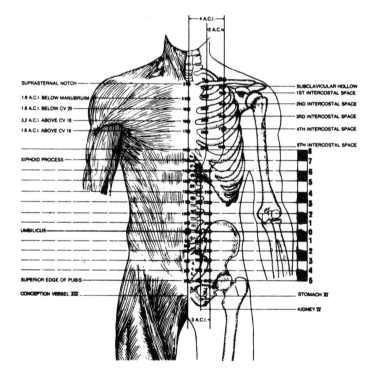

© J.R. Worsley, 1972.

Excerpts from SOPHIA Handbook

To come to life more fully

so as to serve life more wisely

and more nobly

Sagely stillness within

Sovereign service without

Over the years, many patients, in observing the changes that occurred during acupuncture treatment, in themselves and in the lives around them, asked to learn the personal and observational skills of traditional acupuncture. These people, ranging from corporate CEOs to those already in healing professions, did not wish to learn to treat patients with needles or change their occupations. They wanted to become practiced in using the gifts of the five elements and the particular distinctions that are the fruits of Chinese philosophy.

As a result of these requests, SOPHIA—the School of Philosophy and Healing in Action—was created in 1987 through the masterful vision of John Sullivan. Since that time, my colleagues Jack Daniel, Bob Duggan, Julia Measures, John Sullivan and I have worked together to teach SOPHIA students how to take effective action in being practitioners for life.

The following pages are excerpts from the handbook created through the particular efforts of Julia Measures for use in SOPHIA. In including them, it is my intention that these distinctions open up new possibilities for us all in using the god-given gifts to see, to hear, to ask, to feel. Let these pages serve as a springboard for fresh inquiry into serving life in the dance of the five elements.

NUMBERS ONE TO FIVE

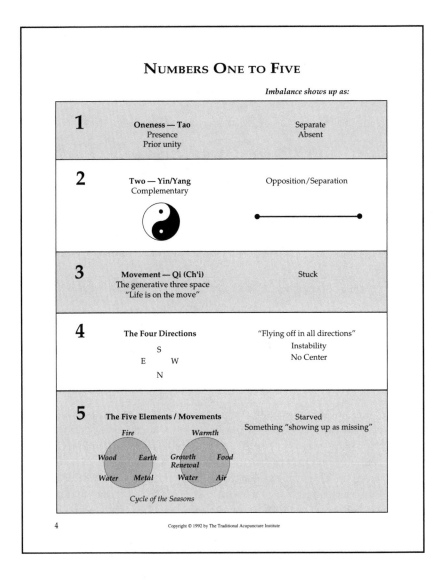

Imbalance shows up as:

1

Oneness — Tao
Presence
Prior unity

Separate
Absent

2

Two — Yin/Yang
Complementary

Opposition/Separation

3

Movement — Qi (Ch'i)
The generative three space
"Life is on the move"

Stuck

4

The Four Directions

S
E   W
N

"Flying off in all directions"
Instability
No Center

5

The Five Elements / Movements

Fire   Warmth
Wood   Earth   Growth   Food
                   Renewal
Water   Metal   Water   Air

Cycle of the Seasons

Starved
Something "showing up as missing"

4

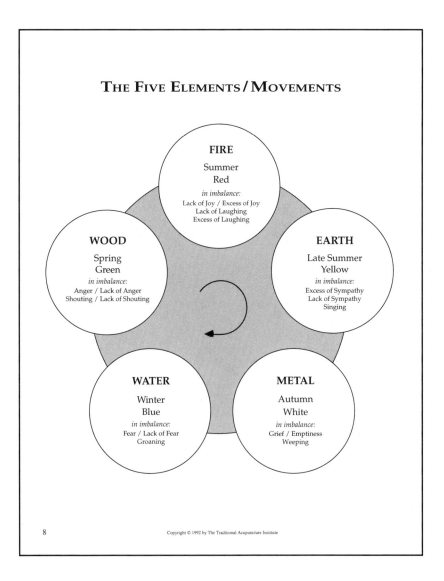

THE FIVE ELEMENTS / MOVEMENTS

FIRE

Summer
Red

in imbalance:
Lack of Joy / Excess of Joy
Lack of Laughing
Excess of Laughing

WOOD

Spring
Green

in imbalance:
Anger / Lack of Anger
Shouting / Lack of Shouting

EARTH

Late Summer
Yellow

in imbalance:
Excess of Sympathy
Lack of Sympathy
Singing

WATER

Winter
Blue

in imbalance:
Fear / Lack of Fear
Groaning

METAL

Autumn
White

in imbalance:
Grief / Emptiness
Weeping

GIFTS FROM THE FIVE MOVEMENTS OF LIFE

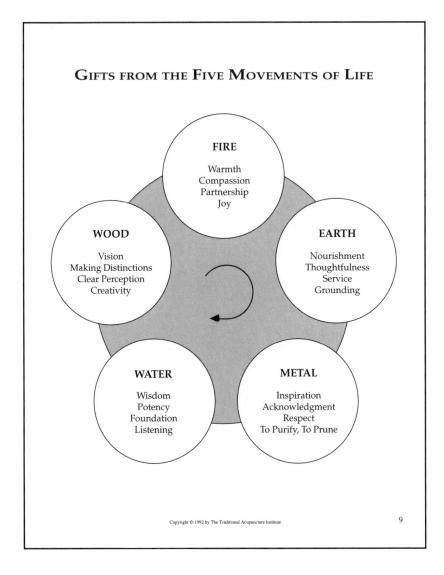

FIRE

Warmth
Compassion
Partnership
Joy

WOOD

Vision
Making Distinctions
Clear Perception
Creativity

EARTH

Nourishment
Thoughtfulness
Service
Grounding

WATER

Wisdom
Potency
Foundation
Listening

METAL

Inspiration
Acknowledgment
Respect
To Purify, To Prune

9

THE INQUIRY INTO A CONCERN — TO COME TO KNOW
To See, To Hear, To Ask, To Feel

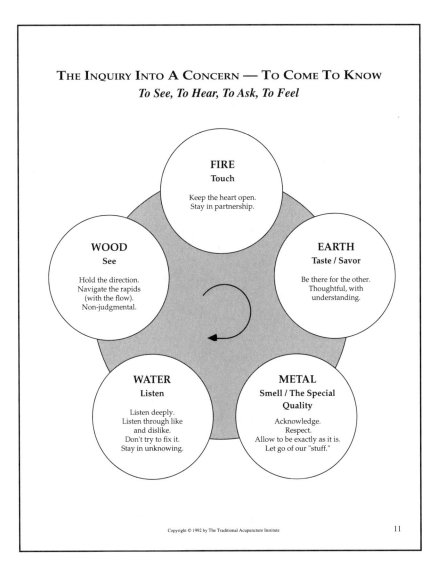

FIRE
Touch

Keep the heart open.
Stay in partnership.

WOOD
See

Hold the direction.
Navigate the rapids
(with the flow).
Non-judgmental.

EARTH
Taste / Savor

Be there for the other.
Thoughtful, with
understanding.

WATER
Listen

Listen deeply.
Listen through like
and dislike.
Don't try to fix it.
Stay in unknowing.

METAL
Smell / The Special
Quality

Acknowledge.
Respect.
Allow to be exactly as it is.
Let go of our "stuff."

11

169

Bibliography

CLASSICS

Nei Ching: The Yellow Emperor's Classic of Internal Medicine.
   Translated by Ilza Veith, University of California Press,
   Berkeley, CA., 1972
The Book of Lieh-Tzu. Translated by A.C. Graham, Ph.D. John
   Murray Publishers, 50 Albemarle, London, 1960
Lao Tzu: Tao Teh Ching. Translated by John C.H. Wu. Edited by
   Paul K.T. Sih. St. John's University Press, NY, 1961

MODERN

Cummings, E.E., *Complete Poems, 1904–1962,* Liveright Publishing
   Corporation, 1991
Kunitz, Stanley, *Passing Thru,* Atlantic Monthly Press
Moon, William Least Heat, *Blue Highways,* Little, Brown and
   Company Publishers, Boston, MA
Needham, Joseph. *Science and Civilization in China.* Vol. II,
   Cambridge University Press, Cambridge, England, 1956
Paz, Octavio, *Configurations,* New Directions Publishing
   Corporation. 1971
Porkert, Manfred. *Theorectical Foundations of Chinese
   Medicine: Systems of Correspondence.* The MIT Press,
   Cambridge, MA, 1974
Scott-Maxwell, Florida, *The Measure of My Days,* Random
   House, New York, NY, 1986
Worsley, J.R. *Is Acupuncture for You?,* Harper & Row, NY, 1973
   The Law of the Five Elements (Chart) Acupuncture, 1972
   The Meridians of Ch'i Energy (4 Charts) Acupuncture,
      Leamington Spa, UK, 1972
   The Acupuncturist's Therapeutic Pocket Book, The Centre
      for Traditional Acupuncture, Columbia, MD, 1975
      (out of print)
   Class notes accumulated during the period from 1971 to 1975

Notes

Complete bibliographic information is found on p. 170. The abbreviation NC has been used for the *Nei Ching*.

Chapter One—INTRODUCTION TO THE FIVE ELEMENTS

1. NC p. 136; 2. NC p. 10; 3. NC p. 152; 4. Needham p. 76; 5. Lao Tzu p. 93; 6. Lao Tzu p. 29; 7. Lao Tzu p. 7; 8. Lieh-Tzu p. 7; 9. NC p. 198; 10. Lieh-Tzu p. 7; 11. NC p. 149.

Chapter Two—WOOD

1. NC p. 144; 2. NC p. 154; 3. NC p. 125; 4. NC p. 102; 5. NC p. 137; 6. NC p. 175; 7. NC p. 133; 8. NC p. 118; 9. NC p. 147; 10. NC p. 109; 11. NC p. 199; 12. NC p. 201; 13. NC p. 23; 14. NC p. 141; 15. Needham p. 244; 16. NC p. 34; 17. NC p. 207; 18. NC p. 222; 19. NC p. 169; 20. NC p. 139; 21. NC p. 140; 22. NC p. 118; 23. NC p. 112; 24. Porkert p. 119; 25. NC p. 123; 26. NC p. 110; 27. NC p. 108; 28. NC p. 107; 29. NC p. 139; 30. NC p. 208; 31. NC p. 15; 32. NC p. 222; 33. NC p. 215; 34. Porkert p. 121; 35. Porkert p. 153; 36. NC p. 206; 37. NC p. 206; 38. NC p. 175; 39. NC p. 124.

Chapter Three—FIRE

1. NC p. 141; 2. NC p. 154; 3. NC p. 102; 4. NC p. 175; 5. NC p. 110; 6. Porkert p. 127; 7. Worsley classroom lectures; 8. NC p. 133; 9. NC p. 133; 10. NC p. 133; 11. NC p. 104; 12. NC p. 226; 13. NC pp. 118–119; 14. NC p. 147; 15. NC p. 148; 16. NC p. 141; 17. NC p. 23; 18. Needham p. 245; 19. NC p. 112; 20. NC p. 119; 21. NC p. 207; 22. NC p. 111; 23. NC p. 107; 24. NC p. 242; 25. NC p. 196; 26. NC p. 122; 27. NC p. 169; 28. NC p. 140; 29. NC p. 119; 30. NC p. 207; 31. NC p. 243; 32. NC p. 189; 33. NC p. 139; 34. NC p. 208; 35. Porkert p. 127; 36. Porkert p. 127; 37. NC p. 162; 38. NC p. 143; 39. NC p. 203; 40. NC p. 209; 41. NC p. 184; 42. NC p. 176; 43. NC p. 173; 44. NC p. 163.

Chapter Four—EARTH

1. NC p. 141; 2. NC p. 148; 3. NC p. 184; 4. NC p. 133; 5. NC p. 146; 6. Needham p. 244; 7. NC p. 140; 8. NC p. 169; 9. Porkert p. 131; 10. Porkert p. 133; 11. NC p. 169.

Chapter Five—METAL

1. NC p. 141; 2. NC p. 102; 3. NC p. 176; 4. NC p. 133; 5. Porkert p. 139; 6. NC p. 147; 7. Needham p. 244; 8. NC p. 141; 9. NC p. 207; 10. NC p. 200; 11. NC p. 119; 12. NC p. 120; 13. NC p. 140; 14. NC p. 120; 15. NC p. 208; 16. Porkert p. 139; 17. Porkert p. 156; 18. NC p. 165.

Chapter Six—WATER

1. NC p. 141; 2. NC p. 177; 3. NC p. 103; 4. NC p. 133; 5. Porkert p. 146; 6. NC p. 205; 7. NC p. 133; 8. NC p. 148; 9. Needham p. 244; 10. NC p. 147; 11. NC p. 206; 12. NC p. 120; 13. NC p. 170; 14. NC p. 208; 15. NC p. 139; 16. Porkert p. 144; 17. Porkert p. 156; 18. NC p. 183; 19. NC p. 174; 20. NC p. 209.

Chapter Seven—TRADITIONAL EXAMINATION

1. NC p. 163; 2. NC p. 42; 3. NC p. 159; 4. NC p. 173; 5. NC p. 150; 6. NC p. 118.

Chapter Eight—TRADITIONAL DIAGNOSIS AND TREATMENT

1. The clinical material in this section comes from my files at the Acupuncture Clinic of the College of Chinese Acupuncture, Oaken Holt, Farmoor, Oxford, UK. Facts have been somewhat altered to protect identity.
2. NC p. 184; 3. Porkert p. XIV; 4. NC p. 157; 5. NC p. 224; 6. NC p. 124; 7. NC p. 150; 8. NC p. 226; 9. NC p. 97; 10. NC p. 152; 11. NC p. 154; 12. NC p. 248.

Index

A

Abdomen Sorrow, 59
Abundant Reservoir, 59
Acupuncture, bad, consequences, 120
Acupuncture, Chinese College of, 2, 5
Acupuncture in its anaesthetic use, 3
Acupuncture, symptomatic, 3, 41
Acupuncture, Traditional, 3, 4, 15, 91-92
Acupuncture, Traditional, examination, 89
Acupuncture, Traditional, experience of, 2
Aggressive Energy, 117
Akabane, 105, 106
Alarm points, 103
Ambition, 82
Anger, 26
Anus, 79
Artemesia, 78
Artemisia vulgaris latiflora, 118
Ashen, 35
Ask, to, 107
Autumn, 64

B

Balance, 5
Balance within each meridian, law of, 118
Barefoot doctor, 3
Bitter, 39, 40
Birth, age, date, time and place, 90
Bladder, 14, 38, 76, 78, 81, 82, 83, 93, 94, 100, 101, 102, 104, 105
Blazing Valley, 84
Blood Vessels, 42
Blue, 76
Body clock, 23, 94, 105
Body Mind Spirit, 5, 15, 21, 31, 36
Bone marrow, 81
Bones, 81, 97
Bowels, 97
Bubbling Spring, 84
Burning Spaces, 38

C

Capacity for belching, 57
Capacity for control, 27
Capacity for sadness and grief, 43
Capacity to cough, 68
Capacity to create trembling, 81
Causative factor, 89, 113
Center, 53
Ch'i Cave, 84

Ch'i energy, 3, 4, 5, 11, 12, 13, 14, 21, 22, 26, 27, 29, 35, 46, 47, 59, 69, 70, 83, 84, 100, 111, 1 12 ,118, 122
Ch'i Po, iv, 14, 24, 28, 46, 105, 121
Ch'i Rushing, 59
Chou, Lower, 38, 104
Chou, Middle, 38, 104
Chou, Upper, 38, 104
Circulation Sex, 36, 37, 38, 39, 40, 42, 45, 46, 47, 94, 1 00, 101, 102, 104, 113
Classics, 44
Climate, 27, 43, 58, 69, 78, 94
Cloud Gate, 70
Cold, 78
Color, 22, 35, 52, 64, 76
Color, favorite, 93
Complexion, 43
Conception Vessel, 103, 104
Control Cycle, of Energy, 117
Correspondences, 16-17, 25, 27, 29, 44, 58, 70, 82, 111
Cure, Law of, 92
Cures, one-needle, 121
Cycle of life, 11
Cycle of the seasons, 11, 120

D

Dampness, 58
Dark Gate, 84
Decision maker, 37
Diagnosis, 3, 4, 5, 11, 24, 25, 26, 29, 31, 47, 87, 100, 105, 107, 117
Diagnosis, abdominal, 103
Diagnosis, pulse, 4, 11
Diagnosis, Traditional, 111-114
Diagnosis, Traditional, process, 107
Diagnostic tools, 22
Diet, 99
Direction, 24, 39, 53, 66, 78
Disease, destructive, 117
Dizzy, 95
Dooley, Dr. Thomas, 1
Drainer of the Dregs, 65
Dreams, 28, 44, 58, 69, 82, 98
Drink, 98
Dryness, 69
Dust Bin Collector, 65

E

Ears, 40, 79, 95
Earth, 14, 51-59, 80, 94, 100, 112, 113 (character, 49)
Earth imbalance, 52, 53, 54, 55, 57, 112, 113
Earth Motivator, 59

Transporter of energy, 54
Treatment, 3, 4, 5, 11, 25, 105, 115-122, 125
Treatment, course, 121
Triple Heater, 38
Triple Warmer, 38

U
Upper Chou, 38, 104
Urethra, 79
Urination, 97

V
Vegetable, 29, 44, 58, 70, 82
Viscera, five, 54
Vital essence, 77, 78
Vital force, 12
Vitals Correspondence, 84

W
Wang Ping, 84
Warmth and maintenance official, 40
Water, 14, 75-84, 96, 98, 99, 100, 105, 113
(character, 73)
Water, imbalance, 75, 78, 79, 80, 81, 97
Way, the, 12
Weeping, 67
Welcome Fragrance, 96
West, 66
White, 64
Wind, 27
Will power, 82
Wind, east, 24
Wind, south, 43
Winter, 76
Wood, 14, 21-31, 51, 94, 95, 97, 116, 117
(character, 19)
Wood, concept of, 21
Wood, imbalance, 23, 24, 25, 27, 106, 116
Wood, out of balance, 21, 99
Worsley, J.R., Professor, 2, 5, 18, 36, 37, 45, 54, 65, 77, 78, 107, 116

Y
Yin Yang, 5, 12, 14, 29, 45, 47
Yellow, 52

For More Information

Dianne Connelly is a co-founder of Tai Sophia Institute (formerly Traditional Acupuncture Institute) which is a tremendous resource for more information on Traditional Acupuncture and the Five Elements.

Visit Tai Sophia's website—www.tai.edu—for more information on the Institute's resources and services, which include:

· Graduate programs in Acupuncture, Botanical Healing, and Applied Healing Arts.

· Community and graduate workshops and seminars. Some of these educational offerings are conducted by Dianne Connelly.

· A bookstore for the healing arts—Meeting Point Bookstore— which offers other Tai Sophia titles, including another by Dianne Connelly.

You can also find out more about Tai Sophia Institute through The Pulse, a free quarterly catalog of workshops, or Meridians, a quarterly magazine ($20 for 4 issues). Dianne Connelly writes a regular column for Meridians. Call 800/735-2968 to request these publications.

For catalog and price list on wholesale orders of this book or other Tai Sophia publications contact:
        Meeting Point Bookstore
        at Tai Sophia Institute
        7750 Montpelier Road
        Laurel, MD 20723
        phone 800/735-2968
        e-mail bookstore@tai.edu

Order Form

Please send me additional copies of Traditional Acupuncture:
The Law of the Five Elements.

Name _____

Address _____

City _____ State _____ Zip _____

Daytime Phone (_____) _____

Number of Copies _____ x $16.00 = $ _____

Shipping & Handling $ _____

Maryland Residents, 5% Sales Tax $ _____

Total Amount Enclosed $ _____

Shipping and Handling: $5.00 for the first book and $1.00 each
additional.

❑   I have enclosed a check for the above amount.
❑   Please charge on my ❑ VISA ❑ Mastercard

Card Number _____ Exp. Date _____

Signature _____

Mail order form to Meeting Point Bookstore, Tai Sophia
Institute, 7750 Montpelier Road, Laurel, Maryland 20723